Periodontal Therapy

Periodontal Therapy

Claude L. Nabers, D.D.S.
Past President
American Academy of Periodontology
Past Chairman
American Board of Periodontology
San Antonio, Texas

William H. Stalker, D.D.S.
Private Practice
Diplomate, American Board of Periodontology
San Antonio, Texas

1990
B.C. DECKER, Inc. • Toronto • Philadelphia

Publisher

B.C. Decker Inc
3228 South Service Road
Burlington, Ontario   L7N 3H8

B.C. Decker Inc
320 Walnut Street
Suite 400
Philadelphia, Pennsylvania   19106

Sales and Distribution

United States and Puerto Rico
The C.V. Mosby Company
11830 Westline Industrial Drive
Saint Louis, Missouri   63146

Canada
McAinsh & Co. Ltd.
2700 Old Leslie Street
Willowdale, Ontario   M2K 2X5

Australia
McGraw-Hill Book Company Australia Pty. Ltd.
4 Barcoo Street
Roseville East 2069
New South Wales, Australia

Brazil
Editora McGraw-Hill do Brasil, Ltda.
rua Tabapua, 1.105, Itaim-Bibi
Sao Paulo, S.P. Brasil

Colombia
Interamericana/McGraw-Hill de Colombia, S.A.
Apartado Aereo 81078
Bogota, D.E. Colombia

Europe
McGraw-Hill Book Company GmbH
Lademannbogen 136
D-2000 Hamburg 63
West Germany

France
MEDSI/McGraw-Hill
6, avenue Daniel Lesueur
75007 Paris, France

Hong Kong and China
McGraw-Hill Book Company
Suite 618, Ocean Centre
5 Canton Road
Tsimshatsui, Kowloon
Hong Kong

India
Tata McGraw-Hill Publishing Company, Ltd.
12/4 Asaf Ali Road, 3rd Floor
New Delhi 110002, India

Indonesia
P.O. Box 122/JAT
Jakarta, 1300 Indonesia

Italy
McGraw-Hill Libri Italia, s.r.l.
Piazza Emilia, 5
I-20129 Milano MI
Italy

Japan
Igaku-Shoin Ltd.
Tokyo International P.O. Box 5063
1-28-36 Hongo, Bunkyo-ku,
Tokyo 113, Japan

Korea
C.P.O. Box 10583
Seoul, Korea

Malaysia
No. 8 Jalan SS 7/6B
Kelana Jaya
47301 Petaling Jaya
Selangor, Malaysia

Mexico
Interamericana/McGraw-Hill de Mexico, S.A. de C.V.
Cedro 512, Colonia Atlampa
(Apartado Postal 26370)
06450 Mexico, D.F., Mexico

New Zealand
McGraw-Hill Book Co. New Zealand Ltd.
5 Joval Place, Wiri
Manukau City, New Zealand

Panama
Editorial McGraw-Hill Latinoamericana, S.A.
Apartado Postal 2036
Zona Libre de Colon
Colon, Republica de Panama

Portugal
Editora McGraw Hill do Portugal, Ltda.
Rua Rosa Damasceno 11A–B
1900 Lisboa, Portugal

South Africa
Libriger Book Distributors
Warehouse Number 8
"Die Ou Looiery"
Tannery Road
Hamilton, Bloemfontein 9300

Southeast Asia
McGraw-Hill Book Co.
348 Jalan Boon Lay
Jurong, Singapore 2261

Spain
McGraw-Hill/Interamericana de Espana, S.A.
Manuel Ferrero, 13
28020 Madrid, Spain

Taiwan
P.O. Box 87–601
Taipei, Taiwan

Thailand
632/5 Phaholyothin Road
Sapan Kwai
Bangkok 10400
Thailand

United Kingdom, Middle East and Africa
McGraw-Hill Book Company (U.K.) Ltd.
Shoppenhangers Road
Maidenhead, Berkshire
SL6 2QL England

Venezuela
McGraw-Hill/Interamericana, C.A.
2da. calle Bello Monte
(entre avenida Casanova y Sabana Grande)
Apartado Aereo 50785
Caracas 1050, Venezuela

Periodontal Therapy

ISBN 1–55664–219–9

Library of Congress catalog card number: 89-51246

10 9 8 7 6 5 4 3 2 1

Preface

The successful dentist of the 1990s will have periodontics at the core of his (or her) practice. Nevertheless, although many outstanding textbooks on periodontics exist, none addresses the need to incorporate periodontics into the private practice environment. *Periodontal Therapy* was developed to fill that void.

In an era in which fluoride has eliminated much of the need for restorative dentistry, today's dentist must expand his area of expertise to stay busy. The dentist must be capable of evaluating the many new periodontal therapies that are constantly being introduced so that he does not incorporate ineffective therapies into his practice. Today's patient is more aware of periodontal disease, and failure to diagnose periodontal disease is now one of the leading causes of litigation in dentistry.

Periodontal Therapy is designed above all to be a practical guide for the dentist in private clinical practice. It therefore presents the indications, objectives, and techniques for all proven clinical procedures in a format that follows current ADA and insurance company procedural codes. Our goal has been to simplify the process of identifying problems and selecting the best and least traumatic treatment options available.

Periodontal Therapy also discusses in detail the other major challenges that we face in daily practice: patient motivation, dentistry in an age of litigation, and the problems of AIDS and herpes.

The sections on patient evaluation and motivation will be especially helpful: We all know that the primary obstacle we face in private practice today is patient reluctance to seek and accept treatment. Motivation is as important as quality of service in promoting patient satisfaction—and a satisfied patient is our best source of reference.

Periodontal Therapy contains contributions from some of the outstanding periodontists in America today, along with a wealth of clinical photographs and techniques. In it we present the distillation of almost 50 years of experience gained in daily clinical practice.

Claude L. Nabers
William H. Stalker

Contents

Periodontal Therapy

CHAPTER ONE

Patient Evaluation and Motivation

The successful and busy dentist of the 90's will have preventive dentistry and periodontal therapy as the mainstay of his (or her) practice. To implement these vital services, the dentist must understand what each patient wants and expects from any indicated dental procedures. Any dentist who wants to be truly successful in the long term must establish goals or "game plans" for his professional as well as his personal life. One element in any such plan must be establishing a good working relationship with patients right from the first encounter. The ability to size up a patient's personality early in your relationship—is this patient likely to be stoical, sensitive to pain, easily offended, and so on—is an important skill. Motivating the patient to pursue necessary programs of dental therapy, follow instructions, and pay bills is also part of your professional role.

Meeting the Patient

Always greet each new patient by name and welcome him (or her) into your practice. Always shake hands as you greet the patient, and take note of the type of handshake. Moisture can indicate nervousness. Firmness can indicate dominance level. Notice, too, whether the patient looks you in the eye or glances away. This will give you some insight into the patient's self-confidence. Look, listen, and ask questions as you talk with new patients. Instruct your secretary to make an early appointment with each new patient for a short, cursory examination, and tell the patient that this examination will be a short one. Find out what the patient's chief complaint is when he arrives, and have him fill out a medical and dental history questionnaire if there is time before he is to be seen. Otherwise, have the patient fill out the forms at the end of the cursory examination. At this examination, perform the O'Leary periodontal screening examination as described in Chapter 2. From your short examination, you should know if the patient is a candidate for emergency care for existing pain, or if there is a need for a thorough caries or periodontal examination, full mouth x-ray studies, occlusal evaluation with mounted casts, or referral to someone else who could better care for them. This short examination should only take 10 minutes, and you can then decide which course to follow.

Periodontal therapy is completely successful only when the patient understands both his problems and the treatment required. It may be that the patient is not one whom you wish to treat. In that case, do not charge the patient for this appointment and refer him (or her) elsewhere. Tell him that his problems are outside the scope of your practice but you will help him find the best doctor for his problems.

Evaluating the Patient

Several patient classifications have become part of the folklore of the profession over the years—all of them to be taken with a grain of salt, to be sure, but all containing a kernel of truth.

THE SOMATOTYPE SYSTEM

One classification system, for which I am obliged to Dr. F.M. Black of Fort Worth, Texas, describes patients in terms of somatotypes. The vast majority of patients, according to Dr. Black, can be understood as having characteristics from one or two of the following categories:

1. The Endomorph. This patient is pear-shaped, with heavy arms and legs. He (or she) tends to be late for appointments. His teeth are important to him, he says, because he needs them to chew. If you need to get him to start talking, ask him if he's been to any good new restaurants recently. Once he's told that dentures will probably chew only about 12% as well as his own teeth, you'll have his complete cooperation in a thorough dentistry program.
2. The Mesomorph. Athletic, a go-getter, this patient is prompt and likes to be recognized. *Don't keep him (or her) waiting!* Arrange your schedule so that he can be first in the morning or afternoon, and tell him you're allotting him this special time to lessen the chance of having an emergency disrupt the appointment. Don't ever be late for this patient.
3. The Ectomorph. This patient is more serious, not particularly athletic, and interested in learning new things. Be sure to tell him (or her) about all the modern high-tech procedures you plan to use in his care.

THE EMOTIONAL NEED SYSTEM

Another popular classification system is one put forward many years ago by Roy Garn. In this system, people are categorized in terms of their emotional needs. Garn suggested the following stereotypes:

1. The Recognition Person. This patient loves recognition and will spend time, effort, and money—in short, will do anything needed—to get it. This patient is easy to recognize, for, if you let him, he will tell you that he is, was, or is about to become President of this, that, or the other. If you want him as a lifelong admirer, cut out newspaper items about him and send them with a personal note or put them in his records so you can give them to him at his next appointment. He is already aware of the importance of appearance in creating a good first impression, and when you tell him that he needs his teeth more than 99% of your patients, you're only confirming what he already believes. Knowing this, you can motivate him (or her) to appreciate the need to have his own teeth. The teeth are vital to a healthy, happy, and friendly appearance, and he needs them for enunciation as well as for chewing. Has he ever heard someone with whistling or chattering dentures?

2. The Self-Preservationist. This patient will do everything possible to have the longest, healthiest, and most robust life possible. He jogs, doesn't smoke or drink, gets a good night's sleep every night, and never gets fat. He knows a lot about nutrition and diet and follows physicians' orders scrupulously. To gain this patient's cooperation, let him know that dental infections release showers of bacteria into the bloodstream. Show him the bacterial activity from his plaque with a phase-contrast or darkfield microscope. Discuss with him why a good preventive program is at the heart of modern dentistry.

3. The Romance Person. This patient is extremely concerned with his (or, again, her) appearance. He likes all the good things money can buy, like cars, suits, dresses, jewelry—and beautiful teeth. He's a sharp dresser, and he likes to be complimented on the fact. (The feminine version does an outstanding job on her makeup, sometimes starves herself to stay in shape, and loves honest compliments.) This patient is not so much interested in discussing chewing or health, but needs only to be aware of how important the teeth are to smiles, facial contours, and beauty.

4. The Money Person. This person wants to know how much his treatment will cost before you've even formulated a diagnosis. Regardless of the type of treatment needed, tell him he's lucky to catch the problem this early: treatment will be shorter and less costly if begun *now*. He may be extremely wealthy, but he must be convinced that he will actually save money by having preventive and corrective periodontal treatment now rather than later.

THE DOMINANCE SYSTEM

Another classification system is based on dominance level. This system makes use of three stereotypes:

1. The Extremely Dominant Person. This patient is really an extrovert bully. He (or occasionally she) doesn't sit in the chair when shown into the dentist's office. When the dentist arrives, he's usually standing up, looking at his x-rays on the viewbox or checking his watch. He is not a good listener

and doesn't like to be told what to do. So, how can you motivate him? Lead him to tell *you* what should be done. For example, you can show him the pockets, the pus, the looseness of his teeth, and so on. Then ask him what he would do if he had an apple that had a rotten spot on it but was otherwise good. He will answer firmly, "Cut the bad part out." He has just told you what to do with any pockets that remain after scaling, root planing, and oral hygiene procedures have been done. Tell this patient that the bad tissue may be scraped away in some areas, cut away in other areas, or flapped and grafted into a new and better position. Do not confuse him by going into great detail.

2. The Moderately Dominant Person. You can communicate more easily with this patient, and he (or she) is much more receptive to being educated about his problems, treatment needs, and so on. You should, however, also have this patient tell you how to eliminate the bad area on the apple.

3. The Low-Dominance Person. This patient is extremely quiet, very reserved, and introverted. He (or she) rarely looks you in the eye and speaks very softly. Do not ask him to make any decisions on treatment. Instead, guide, direct, and lead him at all times. Always tell him what his problems are, and reassure him that treatment is available and that you will care for these needs and do your very best for him. As with all patients, make sure he understands that his home treatments are essential for long-term success.

THE PANKEY SYSTEM

Yet another classification system is that developed by Dr. L.D. Pankey, an astute observer of human nature and a master communicator. Dr. Pankey's classification is as follows:

1. The Class I Patient. This patient has a high dental IQ, appreciates good dentistry, and can afford any fair fee. Alas, not all patients fit this description. Many, however, can be elevated to this category by education and proper motivation.

2. The Class II Patient. This patient has a good dental IQ and a desire for good dentistry, but also has some difficulty in paying for it. He (or she) will make an excellent patient if given an opportunity to pay his bill on a deferred budget plan. A specific arrangement and signed papers are indicated if this is to be a happy business arrangement. This includes getting pretreatment estimates on insurance payments.

3. The Class III Patient. This patient does not have a good dental IQ but can afford good dentistry. This patient should be carefully educated in order to be reclassifed as a Class I or Class II patient. Never talk this patient into major dental procedures without first getting his dental IQ to the point that he can appreciate your hard work and pay for it with gratitude.

4. The Class IV Patient. This patient has a very low dental IQ and cannot afford any fee. He usually seeks emergency care for pain relief and may even have obviously missing teeth and not be bothered about it at all. He may not seek help until acute necrotizing ulcerative gingivitis (ANUG) has developed. He rarely returns after pain has been eliminated, often does not pay his bill, and frequently has to be turned in for collection.

Patient Motivation

There are many factors to consider in your dealings with patients.

1. When talking with a patient, always start by addressing him (or her) by name. People like to hear their name spoken. It will get their attention to start with, and then they will hear what you have to say.
2. Use the word "thorough" frequently. For example say, "I am sorry to take so long, but we want to do a thorough job." Or, "You are doing a thorough and effective job in your plaque control on most surfaces of your teeth. Let me show you where you can still improve."
3. If you are right-handed, ask the patient to raise his left hand when he wants you to stop at any time. When you have had his mouth open for 1 to 2 minutes, say "you haven't raised your hand yet—are you doing OK?" At least every 5 minutes ask the patient to close and rest his jaws and ask, "How are you doing?" You are programming him to take pride in his ability to cooperate—to keep his mouth open—to not complain, and so on. Praise the patient if he reacts in this way.
4. When you are doing your detailed probe examination, explain to the patient that you are going to measure the crevices around his teeth and that a depth of 1 to 3 mm is normal, that 4 to 5 mm is moderate pocketing, and that 6 mm or deeper indicates severe trouble. Start on the tongue side of the upper left last tooth and call out the numbers to your assistant. When you find a decayed area with your explorer, describe it in lay terms, such as, "There is a soft decayed area between the old filling and the tooth on the third tooth from the back on the tongue side." When you have finished your examination, the patient already knows that he has real problems. If, on the other hand, you have not properly prepared the patient to be an informed third-party listener, he will usually react when told that he has serious problems by saying something like, "What do you mean I have a lot of trouble—it doesn't hurt."

Periodontal Explanations for Patients

Patients must be given answers to the following questions before corrective periodontal treatments start.

1. Where are the periodontal problems and what are they?
2. What caused the problems?
3. What is the best treatment available?
4. How can the results of corrective treatment be maintained?
5. What will be done to prevent discomfort?
6. How many appointments are needed and how long will they be?
7. What will be the total cost (investment for treatments)?

Most patients only want detailed answers to the last three questions.

There are many good patient-education booklets on periodontal diseases. Get the American Academy of Periodontology list of booklets and order the *Journal of Periodontology*.

The following information is for the patient who wants to know the details about his problems and his required therapy. Use any part of it, as well as any other facts you feel are relevant to make your own patient instructional brochure on "Periodontal Diseases." Have it printed with your name, address, and telephone number. Patients who become your missionaires are your best source of reference.

Information on periodontal diseases for patients

The diseases of the dental foundation (diseased gums, jaw-bone destruction, or looseness of teeth) rarely cause pain. When a patient finds out about his periodontal disease in time for corrective treatment to be performed, he is fortunate.

A recent study by the National Institute of Dental Research has shown that the dental health of Americans is better than previously thought. Improved treatment procedures as well as better preventive patient care is probably the reason for this improvement. Almost all of those surveyed had been to a dentist within the last 12 months. Nevertheless, prevention and treatment of periodontal diseases remains of great importance. About 8% of working Americans under 65 years of age have a loss of attachment (tooth support) of 6 millimeters or more in one or more sites. Of those over 65 years of age, 34% suffer from periodontal disease (defined as 6 millimeters or more of attachment loss at one or more sites—one millimeter is about ½₅ inch).

Among those under 65 years of age, 4.2% had no teeth, 45% had gingivitis, and 75% had some evidence of attachment loss. Among those over 65 years of age, 42% had no teeth and 95% showed attachment loss.

If you have a dental foundation problem and are carrying an infection in your mouth that is a continued source of bacteria that can in time cause destruction of teeth, gums, and bone. Timely treatment can restore and maintain a healthy supporting foundation for the teeth so that chewing and talking feel and appear as natural and comfortable as possible. In addition, it will eliminate a source of infection that can threaten your general health.

How can a successful treatment result be obtained? By the following steps:

1. Establishing an accurate diagnosis. An accurate periodontal diagnosis cannot be made until all pertinent information is obtained. Such data can help reveal causative factors, duration of disease, probable outcome for individual teeth and arches, and the treatments needed. Requirements for fillings, root canals and bridgework must also be included in your total dental and periodontal diagnosis and treatment plan.

2. Improving general health. If signs of medical problems are detected, you will be asked to consult your family physician. Periodontal corrective treatments cannot be totally successful unless you are in good health. As health is a relative matter, how you feel is not always a good indication of how healthy you are. Poor diet, underlying systemic diseases, excessive drinking of alcohol, or emotional problems are severe complicating factors for periodontal treatments.

3. Eliminating causative factors. Lasting results can only be obtained when the causative factors are eliminated or controlled. In rare cases, some causative factor may not become known until much later. An example would be unconscious teeth-grinding while sleeping or some medical problem that cannot be detected at the beginning of treatment. Among

the causative factors often found during diagnosis are bacterial growth on the teeth, retention of food particles between the teeth, faulty or worn-out fillings that hold plaque, pockets between the teeth and gums, deformities in the jaw bone around teeth following bone destruction, faulty diet, medical problems that influence all tissues in the body, excessive pressures on the teeth, and missing teeth.

4. Reshaping gums and bone to normal contours and functions. Deviations from normal, such as pockets between teeth and gums or bone defects that result from periodontal diseases, must be treated to achieve long-term periodontal health. Pockets harbor bacteria, causing pus to form. As the pockets go deeper, bone is destroyed.

5. Restoring tooth-to-tooth bracing within the jaws. Missing teeth, open spaces between the teeth, or worn-out fillings may require crowns, bridges, or new fillings to return the jaw arch back to a solid state where the teeth act together and brace each other. After a diagnosis has been made, any need for such work will be explained to you. Sometimes teeth are treated even though the outcome may be doubtful. You will be informed if any of your teeth have an uncertain prognosis.

6. Eliminating or reducing excessive pressures on teeth. The chewing muscles and the teeth should work harmoniously together. If they do not, then the bite of the teeth may need changing. In other words, if the bite is off, so that a tooth strikes too hard, causing bone destruction or looseness of the tooth, the occlusion (the bite of your teeth) must be adjusted. Several or all of the teeth may be involved. Sometimes people who grit or grind their teeth in their sleep need an appliance that can be worn during sleep. Remember, teeth that have been loosened by heavy pressures will usually be lost if not tightened with treatment.

7. Follow-up recall treatments. Follow-up treatments every 3 to 6 months are essential to preserve the results obtained by corrective treatments. As part of your initial corrective periodontal treatments, you will be taught to care for your mouth at home. These home treatments are your best insurance in preventing recurrence of local disease. If you have a need for periodontal treatments, you should know that you are susceptible to future problems, and will need periodic follow-up treatments to correct any beginning problems. For example, inflammation of the gums can lead to bone destruction and pockets. We know that gum inflammation is caused by local irritants. We also know that only your care can prevent local irritants. Unfortunately, though, home care procedures cannot do a perfect job. Therefore, periodic follow-up treatments are needed to remove any local irritants that your home care has not prevented. At these appointments, areas that have been neglected, as well as any need for further corrective treatments, will be brought to your attention. These preventive maintenance treatments are usually performed by a specialist in this field, the dental hygienist. Any new pockets discovered during these treatments must be treated early.

Periodontal treatment will yield lasting results only with your understanding and willingness to cooperate in order to keep your natural teeth.

Most patients do not need to be persuaded of the value of keeping their own teeth, but perusing a list such as that in Table 1–1 may underline the urgency of good dental care.

Table 1–1 • REASONS FOR KEEPING YOUR TEETH

Physical Health

Infections in your mouth can be detrimental to your general health.

Emotional Health

Talking	People with dentures often whistle and click when they speak because the teeth are so important in enunciation.
Preserving appearance	The presence or absence of teeth directly affects facial contours. When teeth are lost, the gums and bone shrink.
Smiling	Smiles are truly natural-looking only when one has one's natural teeth.
Laughing	Because of the embarrassment that slipping dentures can cause, many denture wearers are afraid to laugh.
Singing, playing an instrument	One's ability to sing or play a musical instrument such as a flute or trumpet may be impaired.

Enjoyment of Food

Chewing	Studies have shown that people can chew only about 12% as well with dentures as they can with their own teeth.
Tasting	Complete dentures cover the roof of the mouth and thereby alter the taste of foods
Feeling	The nerves surrounding your natural teeth tell you if food is soft or crunchy. With dentures, you only feel pressure in the gums.

General Comfort

Gagging	Some people have trouble with gagging when wearing dentures.
Halitosis	Dentures can develop a noticeable odor. Pockets harbor bacteria, produce pus, and cause a foul odor.

Table 1–2 outlines the normal sequence followed in a periodontal care program.

Table 1–2 • USUAL SEQUENCE OF TREATMENT*

1. Extractions of hopelessly involved teeth
2. Temporary bridges (if necessary)
3. Initial preparation
   a. plaque control
   b. scaling
   c. caries control
   d. temporary splinting
4. Corrective periodontal treatments
5. Restorative dentistry
6. Occlusal restoration or reconstruction
7. Periodic maintenance and corrective treatments
8. Treatment of any isolated new pockets that may develop
9. Maintenance of occlusal reconstruction

*This is a general outline. In any particular case only some of these procedures will be necessary.

Bibliography

Nabers CL. Periodontal information for patients. Texas Dent J 1965; 83(9):18–19.

Pankey LD, Davis WJ. A philosophy of the practice of dentistry. Toledo: Medical College Toledo, Ohio Press, 1985.

Shirley JL. Body Watchin' Is Fun! Dallas: Group Dynamics, 1973.

Waldman HB. Who uses the services of periodontists. J Periodontol 1988; 59:326–327.

Oral Health of United States Adults. The national survey of oral health in U.S. employed adults and seniors, 1985–1986: National findings. N.I.H. publication no. 87-2868. Bethesda, MD: U.S. Department of Health and Human Services, Public Health Service, National Institutes of Health, 1987.

CHAPTER TWO

Patient Examination

A thorough questionnaire is the simplest and quickest way to obtain vital information about a patient's medical and dental history. Have the patient fill out a questionnaire such as the one shown in Figure 2–1. Pertinent answers should later be transferred from the questionnaire to the patient's case history chart (Figure 2–2). Review with the patient those items that require more detailed information. If the patient has not had a complete medical evaluation recently or has any symptoms of any medical problem, request a medical report with blood chemistries from the patient's physician.

Cursory Examination

A short cursory examination for new patients takes only a few minutes and is an excellent way to develop rapport. When the patient is examined, tell him he may not understand some of the data you dictate to your assistant as you check his teeth and oral tissues. Start by doing an examination of lips, cheeks, tongue, floor of mouth, and palate, and then examine the teeth. Call off healthy-looking tissues and any deviation from normal. Speak in terms the patient can understand: "There is a hole between the old filling on the upper left last molar and the tooth, and it feels soft. The upper left last molar is a little loose when I put pressure on it. There is a redness of the gum between the last two teeth on the upper left."

This is also the time to perform a modified version of the O'Leary screening examination for periodontitis, as described on page 13.

THE FOLLOWING IMPORTANT INFORMATION IS NEEDED TO HELP MAKE YOUR DIAGNOSIS

1. Are you experiencing discomfort from your mouth at this time? _____ Lately? _____

   If so, explain _____

2. How many times have you had your teeth cleaned in the last 5 years? _____ When was the last time? _____

3. Have you had previous periodontal treatments? _____ When? _____ By whom? _____

4. Do your gums ever bleed? _____ When you brush? _____ At night in sleep? _____

5. Have you noticed any loose teeth? _____ Shifting teeth? _____

6. Have you noticed any mouth odors or bad tastes? _____ For how long? _____

7. Have you ever had trench mouth? _____ If so, when? _____

8. Have immediate relatives lost all their natural teeth? _____ Which? _____ Results? _____

9. Are your teeth sensitive to heat, cold, or sweets? _____ Which? _____ For how long? _____

10. Do meats wedge between your teeth? _____ When did you first notice this? _____

11. How often do you brush your teeth? _____ Floss your teeth? _____ Use toothpicks? _____

    Do you use a hard brush? _____ Medium? _____ Soft? _____ Water irrigation devices? _____

12. Do you often have fever blisters on your lips? _____ After dental work? _____

13. Have you had your teeth straightened? _____

14. Would you be tremendously disturbed if you had to lose your teeth and wear false teeth? _____

15. Are you satisfied with the appearance of your teeth? _____

16. Have you been under more nervous tensions than average lately? _____

17. Do you smoke? _____ What and how much? _____

18. Are you aware of grinding your teeth at night in your sleep? _____

    Do you hold your teeth together? _____

19. Do you have clicking? _____ popping? _____ or pain? _____ in jaw joints.

20. Do you have headaches regularly? _____ Mornings? _____ Evenings? _____

    After eating? _____ What do you take for headaches? _____

21. Do you tend to worry or fret about things that do not happen? _____

22. Do you often give up doing things (trips, parties) because of unexpectedly not feeling well? _____

23. Do you consider your medical health to be good? _____ fair? _____ poor? _____

    When was your last check up? _____ By whom? _____

24. Have you ever fainted? _____ In a dental office? _____

25. Are you being treated by a physician at this time? _____ For what? _____

26. Are you taking medicines, drugs, or pills regularly? _____ If so, what? _____

    What medicine works best for you to relieve pain? _____

27. Are you on a diet at this time? _____ Why? _____

28. Have you gained? _____ or lost? _____ weight recently. How much? _____

29. Do you tire easily? _____ Can you briskly walk for 5 blocks? _____

30. HAVE YOU EVER HAD THE FOLLOWING:

Anemia _____	Excessive thirst _____	Bacterial endocarditis _____
Heart disease _____	Liver trouble _____	Severe pain _____
Diabetes _____	Gland trouble _____	Epilepsy _____
Relatives with Diabetes _____	Bladder trouble _____	Need for urination during sleep _____
Hepatitis _____	High blood pressure _____	Are you pregnant? _____
Arthritis _____	Low blood pressure _____	Have you reached menopause? _____
Lung trouble _____	Psychiatric treatment _____	Tuberculosis _____
Gastric Ulcer _____	History of cancer _____	AIDS _____
Duodenal ulcer _____	Excessive bleeding when cut _____	Herpes II _____
Rheumatic fever _____	Clotting problems _____	Other _____
Kidney trouble _____	Venereal disease _____	_____

31. Have you ever taken cortisone? _____ When and for how long? _____ For what? _____

32. Have you ever taken anti coagulants (blood thinner)? _____ If so, when and for how long? _____

33. If you are or ever have been allergic to any medicines or drugs, please indicate which ones by circling? ANTIBIOTICS, ASPIRIN, CODEINE, NOVOCAINE, DEMEROL, PENICILLIN, ANTIHISTAMINES, BARBITURATES. Please list any other allergies _____

34. Have you had major surgery? _____ When? _____ Any complications? _____

35. Do you bruise easily? _____ When did you first notice this? _____

36. Do you normally eat or drink the following daily? Cokes or soft drinks _____ Two vegetables _____ Meat, poultry,

or fish _____ Milk and other dairy products _____ Fruits _____ Eggs _____ Citrus juice _____ Beer _____

Highballs _____ Desserts _____ Candy _____ White bread _____

37. Do you normally eat breakfast? _____ If so, what? _____

38. Have you ever had an extremely frightening experience with dentistry? _____ When? _____

Explain _____

39. Have I treated any of your family or friends? _____ Who? _____

40. Comments: _____

FIGURE 2–1 • Patient questionnaire. In our experience, patients who answer question 14 in the affirmative almost always accept treatment. Patients who give affirmative answers to 22 are more likely to cancel or miss dental appointments.

CASE HISTORY

1. Pain or chief complaint _____

2. Prophys in last 5 years _____

3. Previous Perio. _____

4. Bleeding gingiva _____

5. Loose teeth _____ Shifting teeth _____

6. Bad tastes and odors _____

7. N.U.G. _____

8. F. dentures in family _____

9. Hot, cold, sweet/discomfort _____

10. Open contacts _____

11. _____ Brushes ___/day-Flosses ___/day-Toothpicks _____

Water irrigation devices _____

12. Herpes history _____

13. Orthodontic case _____

14. Disturbed if teeth must be lost _____

15. Likes appearance of teeth _____

16. Nervous tensions _____

17. Smokes _____

18. Occ. habits _____

19. T.M.J. symptoms _____

20. Headaches _____

21. Worries & frets _____

22. Misses trips, parties, (appt's) _____

23. Health _____ Last check-up _____

24. Faints _____ Dental office _____

25. Dr's. care _____

26. Medications _____

_____ Pain _____

27. Diet for _____

28. Weight change _____

29. Tires easily _____ Walk briskly _____

30. Illnesses _____

_____

_____

31. Cortisone _____

32. Anti-coagulants _____

33. Allergies _____

34. Surgery _____

35. Bruise _____

36. Eating habits _____

37. Breakfast _____

38. Fear of dental work _____

39. Friends treated _____

40. Comments: _____

_____

_____

_____

FIGURE 2–2 • Case history form. (This is completed by the assistant and doctor.)

O'Leary Screening Examination

The object of the O'Leary screening examination is to diagnose periodontitis early, before destruction is so advanced that many teeth must be sacrificed. This simple screening examination, which only takes a few minutes, also should be used when examining previously treated patients. Every tooth is examined for gingival status, and the mesial surface of each tooth is then probed for the presence and extent of periodontal pocketing.

ASSESSMENT OF GINGIVAL STATUS

When assessing gingival status, keep in mind the clinical picture of healthy gingiva. Figure 2–3 shows variations in color of healthy gingivae. Darker-pigmented patients have greater pigmentation in the gingiva. Note, however, that in both of the examples shown there is a scalloped contour around each tooth, and the gingival margin is parallel with the cemento-enamel junction. Pointed papillae between the teeth fill the interproximal embrasures, and deflecting contours allow food being masticated to flow away from the teeth. Healthy gingiva is firmly attached to the teeth and to the bone around the teeth.

With a dental mirror to help see all areas, dry the gingival tissues with compressed air and observe any deviations from normal for color, consistency, and evidence of inflammation (Fig. 2–4). Look for ulcerations, spontaneous hemorrhage occurring when the tissue is thoroughly dried with a blast of compressed air, a loss of continuity of any interdental papilla from the buccal to the lingual aspect, and marked deviations from normal contours (enlargement of gingival tissues, recessions exposing root surfaces, or clefts of the gingival tissues). Dictate findings for your assistant to record.

ASSESSMENT OF PERIODONTAL STATUS

Probe the mesial surface of each tooth to determine the presence and extent of periodontal pocketing. It is of the utmost importance that the probe be directed in the long axis of the tooth, as faulty readings result when it is directed at an angle (Fig. 2–5). Probe the surfaces at the mesiofacial line angles and record any depth over 3 mm (Fig. 2–6). The presence of any hemorrhage or exudate on light probing is noted as a presence of disease. Have your assistant mark *H* for hemorrhage and *P* for pus. The mesial method has been found to be about 85% as effective as a thorough examination (i.e., one in which all surfaces on each tooth are probed) in identifying the presence of periodontal disease. If evidence of disease is found, tell the patient and explain that periodontal diseases are the major cause of loss of teeth.

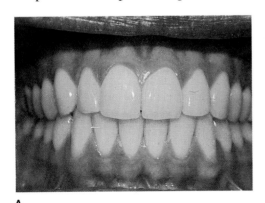 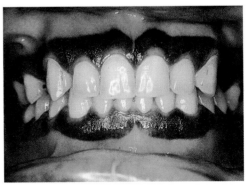

A   B

FIGURE **2–3** • Healthy gingiva. (*A*) In a caucasian. (*B*) In a heavily pigmented patient. Note the variations in the pigmentation of the attached gingiva.

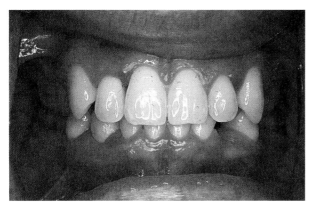

FIGURE **2–4** • Deviations from normal. The marginal tissue is blunted and reddened, the papillae are thickened, and overall the tissues are edematous and swollen.

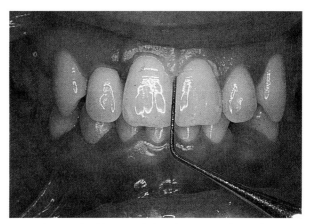

FIGURE **2–5** • Probing mesiofacial crevice of maxillary left central incisor shows a healthy attachment.

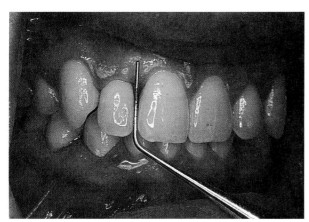

FIGURE **2–6** • Probe placed outside 5-mm pocket on maxillary right lateral incisor. Note bleeding point on mandibular right first premolar canine area.

If the patient has serious problems, is concerned, and desires help, a thorough periodontal examination must be performed to see what problems are present. You can then determine what should be done. If the patient's occlusion shows any deviations from normal, such as centric prematurity or nonfunctional interferences, tell him. If a problem is detected, inform the patient that you will need to make and mount models to study occlusal relationships.

CHARGING FOR THE INITIAL EXAMINATION

To do a thorough periodontal examination, establish a diagnosis, formulate a treatment plan, and explain your treatment takes a minimum of 60 to 90 minutes. It is difficult to charge a patient an adequate fee for this, so establish a fee for this service of only two times your individual overhead cost for the time required for the diagnosis and treatment plan.*

---

*Fees for subsequent therapeutic hourly endeavors should be at least three times your cost of overhead for the time required. Question colleagues on their fee schedules and insurance coverages. Contract total fees should be presented, not individual charges that make up the total cost for treatments.

Oral Clinical Examination Chart
(to be used during examination procedures)

Lymph nodes _____

TMJ tenderness _____

Crepitus _____ Deviation _____

Muscles of mastication _____

Skin _____

Lips _____

Mucous Membrane _____

Tongue _____

Floor of mouth _____

Throat _____

Palate _____

Complete denture prognosis: Max. _____ Mand. _____

Tori: Maxillary _____ Mandibular _____

Gingival color   Pink _____ Red _____

Gingival contours   Good _____ Fair _____ Poor _____

Gingival consistency   Soft _____ Firm _____

Gingival Recession   L _____|_____ R

Erosion   L _____|_____ R

Exudate _____

_____

_____

X-RAY INTERPRETATION

Crown Root Ratio   Good _____ Fair _____ Poor _____

Bone loss   Slight _____ Moderate _____ Advanced _____

Osseous Defects   L _____|_____ R

Decay or Defective Restorations   L _____|_____ R

Other _____

OCCLUSAL ANALYSIS

Over bite _____

Over jet _____

Widest Interincisal Opening _____ MM.

Facets   Slight _____ Moderate _____ Heavy _____

Attrition   Slight _____ Moderate _____ Advanced _____

Buccal — Lingual width   Narrow _____ Medium _____ Broad

Type of Appliance needed _____

_____

_____

Interfering Occlusal Contacts

Centric Relation _____

Right functioning _____

Left functioning _____

Right non-functioning _____

Left non-functioning _____

Protrusive _____

Occlusal sense: Negative _____ Positive _____

Tongue thrust on swallowing _____

LOCAL ETIOLOGICAL FACTORS

Bacterial Plaque _____

Calculus _____

Interproximal food impaction _____

Occlusal Trauma _____

                          DATE |

Blood Pressure _____

FIGURE 2–7 ● Oral clinical examination chart.

Detailed Periodontal Examination

A detailed examination is not needed for simple cases of gingivitis or incipient periodontitis. When there is marked bone loss or tooth mobility due to bone loss or furcation involvements, however, it is essential that you obtain any and all data possible before deciding what you will do. Also, be sure that the patient wants help in keeping his teeth in good health for the maximum period of time. Any patient who is to undergo a major occlusal reconstruction should have a thorough periodontal examination first, and if no pathosis is detected he or she should be started on a preventive program to forestall development of the periodontal disease that often follows major reconstructions.

EXAMINATION PROCEDURES

Ask your assistant, who is to record the findings from your examination (Fig. 2–7), to read each examination procedure and then to record the data you dictate: When asking the patient a question, preface the question with the patient's name. A sample examination procedure follows:

Assistant	Doctor
General Clinical Examination	
Lymph nodes	Check submaxillary, submental, and cervical nodes. Note absence if none are found.
Temporomandibular joints (TMJ)	To patient, while feeling TMJ areas with fingers: "Have you had any clicking, popping, or pain from these joints? Please open wide; now close; now open wide again." Note any deviation to right or left.
Mastication muscles	While feeling temporal muscles, then masseters, ask patient to bite hard on the back teeth. Palpate all muscles of mastication for muscle sensitivity. Dictate developmental status to assistant. (Extremely well-developed muscles of mastication may indicate clenching or grinding habits.)
Skin	To patient: "Have you had any skin problems in the past year or two that have required treatment?" Explain that dermatologic problems can also occur in the mouth. NOTE: Do not hesitate to touch patient's nose, forehead, etc., if any area looks suspicious. Note any flaky keratotic lesions, etc., and ask patient to consult a dermatologist (Figs. 2–8, 2–9).
Lips	List any deviation from normal.
Mucous membranes	After checking all mucous membranes, state findings—white patch at the linea alba, ulcer in cheek, etc. (Fig. 2–10).
Tongue	Hold gauze below lower lip and ask patient to stick his tongue out so you can examine it. After checking dorsal surface of tongue, ask patient to help you. Turn tongue to one side and then the other to check sides and ventral surface (Fig. 2–11). Patients with AIDS often present with hairy leukoplakia on tongue (see Fig. 2–31C).
Floor of the mouth	Retract tongue up with a dental mirror to see if any problems exist and call off findings. NOTE: Watch for keratosis or leukoplakia on the floor of the mouth of heavy smokers (Fig. 2–12).
Throat	Ask patient to stick tongue out. Depress tongue with a dental mirror while asking patient to say "Ah." Be sure to adjust light properly to see down throat. Note any accentuated gag reflexes; if present, tell

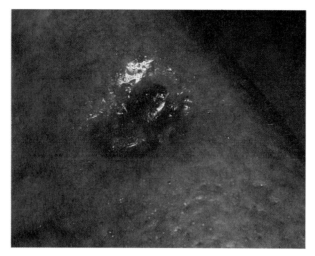

FIGURE 2–8 • Skin lesions. This lesion on the nose was detected at periodontal examination, and the patient was referred to his physician. Diagnosis was carcinoma.

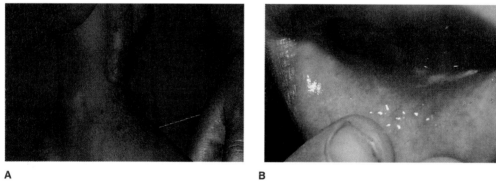

A   B

FIGURE 2–9 • Skin lesions. (A) Typical lesions of hand, foot, and mouth disease (coxsackie virus infection) in a 4-year-old male. (B) Mouth lesion in same patient (patient's finger is in photo).

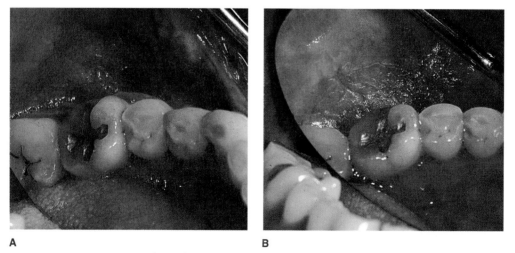

A   B

FIGURE 2–10 • Mucous membrane lesions. (A) Tissue irritation caused by snuff dipping. No biopsy was done. (B) Same area shortly after snuff was discontinued. Ulcerative lesion has resolved.

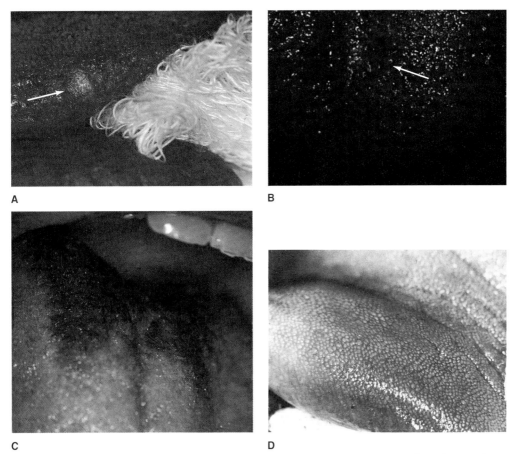

FIGURE 2–11 • Tongue lesions. (A) Smoker's patch on tongue. Patient continued smoking and expired from lung cancer 3 years later. (B) Small lesion detected during periodontal examination. Patient was referred for an excisional biopsy. Diagnosis was malignancy. The patient expired from other causes 15 years later. There was no recurrence of the malignancy. (C) Black hairy tongue. Patient had been on antibiotics for an extended period. (D) Shiny tongue with flattening of the papilla. Therapeutic levels of B-complex supplements will often reverse this phenomenon in a few weeks.

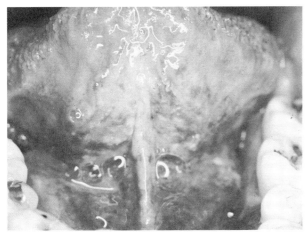

FIGURE 2–12 • Leukoplakia on floor of mouth and ventral of tongue. Biopsy by an oral surgeon led to a histologic diagnosis of dysplasia. Patient continued to smoke and drink heavily. Cancer developed in the same area. Patient died 5 years later, after 2 years of surgical and radiation therapy during which she suffered greatly.

Assistant	Doctor

General Clinical Examination

	patient, "You would hate dentures—the maxillary denture covers the entire hard palate all the way back to the soft palate."
Palate	Using a large palatal mirror, which is approximately three times as large as the dental mirror, check palate for any deviations from normal, such as nicotinic palatinus, ulcers, etc. (Fig. 2–13).
Tori	Feel with your fingers for presence of tori and state findings (Fig. 2–14).
Gingival contours	Visually check buccal and lingual surfaces of all gingival tissues and note if any blunted papillae, gingival craters, etc., are present. Blow compressed air around teeth to detect broken papillae or flapping detached gingiva (see Fig. 2–4).
Gingival consistency	Feel with a blunt instrument to determine if gingival tissues are firm or soft.
Gingival recessions	Note if recession is generalized. Measure any isolated deep areas of recession in millimeters and record for future reference.
Erosions	Note areas of erosion and measure depth of erosion. NOTE: Areas of erosion should not be restored if less than 1.5 mm in depth, carious (rare), or hypersensitive.
Exudate	When probing pockets, note areas with suppurative exudates (pus; marked P) or areas that hemorrhage (marked H) when probed.
Complete denture prognosis	After noting the amounts of attached gingiva and checking for the presence of tori, exostosis, and all other factors influencing the probable ridge quality if all teeth are lost, determine prognosis for full maxillary or full mandibular denture wearing.

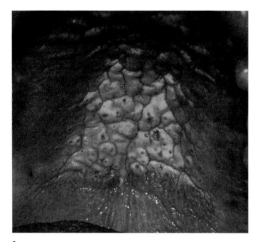
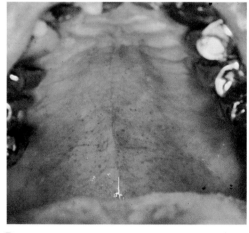

A **B**

FIGURE **2–13** • Lesions of the palate. (A) Nicotinic stomatitis palatinus in a heavy pipe smoker. (B) Minor salivary gland inflammation in a pipe smoker.

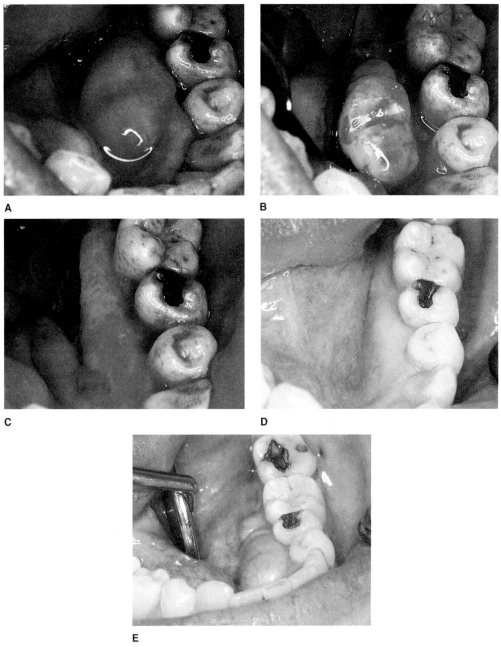

FIGURE 2–14 • Tori. (A) Large mandibular tori. (B) The tori are exposed. (C) The tori have been surgically removed in order to eliminate periodontal pockets. (D) Appearance 3 months after surgery. (E) Same area 15 years later, showing recurrence of tori. The area was not reoperated because pockets had not recurred.

Assistant	Doctor
X-ray Interpretation	
Crown–root ratio	Note length of roots (long, moderately long, etc.). Note any short roots.
Bone loss	Note whether nonexistent, slight, moderate, advanced, or variable from slight to moderate to advanced.

Assistant	Doctor

X-ray Interpretation

Osseous defects	Check x-ray films for evidence of intrabony pockets (Fig. 2–15). Often x-ray studies will not show such defects where probing will. For example, in two-wall interproximal craters the buccal and lingual intact bone shows clearly on x-ray images but interproximal loss of bone will not show. Furca involvements also often fail to show on x-ray studies and can best be determined by furcation probing. It is essential that all radiographic studies be of diagnostic quality using paralleling techniques. Films that are not properly exposed and not of diagnostic quality are useless for periodontal diagnosis and treatment planning. Bone lesions and root structures can be made to appear much larger or smaller than they actually are if the x-ray image is not made parallel to the long axis of the tooth. Additionally, under- or overexposed films mask radiolucent and radiopaque areas that can be important in treatment planning.
Decay or defective restorations	Follow procedure described for cursory examination, using words the patient can understand (Fig. 2–16).
Other observations	Note any possible cysts, periapical abscesses, or suspected rarifying ossifying fibromas that will require vitalometer testing. Also note impacted teeth, dentigerous cysts, internal resorptions, root resorptions, *dens in dente*, periodontal cysts, lack of trabeculation (ground glass appearance, as with hyperparathyroidism), thickened periodontal ligament spaces, or any deviation from normal that may indicate local pathosis or systemic disturbances, etc. (Fig. 2–17).

Occlusal Analysis

Overbite and overjet	Measure overbite and overjet in millimeters using the periodontal probe. This measurement may be needed later to determine occlusal changes. If a night-guard appliance is later required, type will be determined by amount of overbite and overjet.
Widest intercisal opening	Measure (in millimeters or with your fingers) the widest opening patient can comfortably make. If an opening of two or less fingers is recorded, plan on allotting 50% extra time for each appointment because patient will require frequent rests. Also, you should restrict amount of work to be accomplished at each appointment (Fig. 2–18).

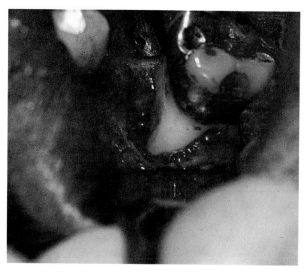

FIGURE **2–15** • Osseous defects. A reflected tissue flap exposes a three-wall osseous defect.

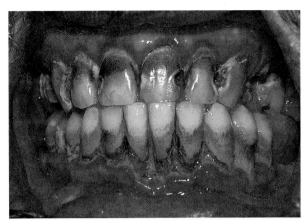

FIGURE **2–16** • Patient showing multiple carious lesions and overall neglect.

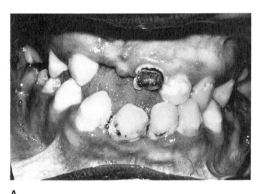

A

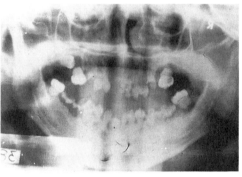

B

FIGURE **2–17** • 20-year-old male with loose teeth. (*A*) Clinical appearance. (*B*) Radiographic appearance. Diagnosis was dentinal dysplasia type II.

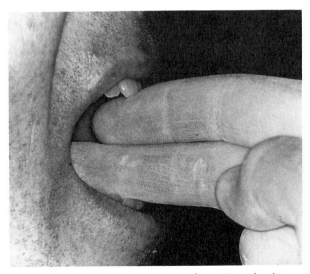

FIGURE **2–18** • Maximum interincisal opening of only two fingers. This may increase later if occlusal prematurities are eliminated.

Assistant	Doctor
Occlusal Analysis	
Facets	Note whether wear is slight, moderate, or advanced. Advanced facet wear patterns suggest bruxism (Fig. 2–19).
Attrition	Note whether attrition is slight, moderate, or advanced.
Buccal-lingual width	Note whether molars are narrow, medium, or broad.
Type of appliance	Note type: None, flat plane night-guard appliance, modified Hawley, Tanner, etc.
Interfering occlusal contacts	Evaluate occlusion on all patients.
Occlusal sense	Ask patient: "Can you chew comfortably on either side of your mouth?" "Do your teeth bite together comfortably?" If either answer

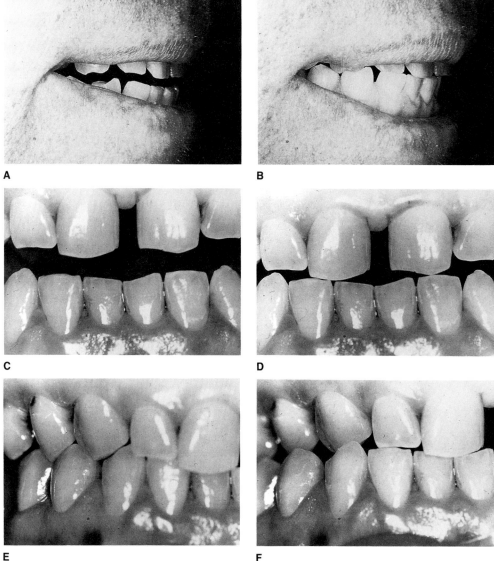

FIGURE 2–19 ● Facet wear patterns. (*A*) Facet wear pattern on canines, indicating history of bruxism. (*B*) Wear facets meshing in extreme right lateral excursion. (*C*) Unusual anterior faceting. (*D*) Protrusive excursion and facets do not match. (*E*) Lateral excursion facets do not match in anterior region. (*F*) Crossover past end-to-end canine relationship shows patient was bruxing in this extreme crossover position. Clinicians should suspect crossover relationships when unusual faceting, mobility and/or periodontal breakdown is apparent on nonfunctional molar teeth.

Assistant	Doctor

Occlusal Analysis

Tongue thrusting on swallowing	is no, then patient has positive occlusal sense. If patient is unaware of having teeth, then he has negative occlusal sense. Holding lips apart, see if tongue thrusts forward when swallowing. Check palatal rugae. If they are flattened out, tongue thrusting is unlikely. If rugae are accentuated, with deep grooves between them, patient is probably a tongue thruster. If teeth have spread apart in recent years and tongue is scalloped on edges and can be seen pushing between teeth when swallowing, then record finding as tongue thrust—heavy (Fig. 2–20). Heavy tongue thrusters will have

FIGURE 2–20 • Tongue thrusting. (A) Anterior open bite. (B) Tongue thrust on swallowing. (C) Accentuated rugae. Tongue thrusters usually have these because they do not have the flattening forces that are generated by tongue pressure in normal glutination. (D) Scalloped tongue contours from excess repeated pressure on the teeth. Patients normally swallow 2000 to 3000 times per day. (E) Orabase and zinc oxide mixture placed on the lateral borders of the tongue prior to having the patient swallow a small amount of water. (F) Orabase and zinc oxide mixture transferred to the lingual surfaces of the maxillary anterior teeth. This is indicative of a myofunctional tongue thrust habit. These patients also have a reduced gag reflex because of excessive uvular stimulation.

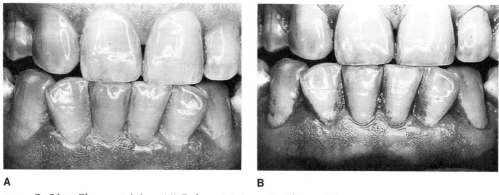

A   **B**

FIGURE 2–21 • Plaque staining. (*A*) Before staining. (*B*) After staining.

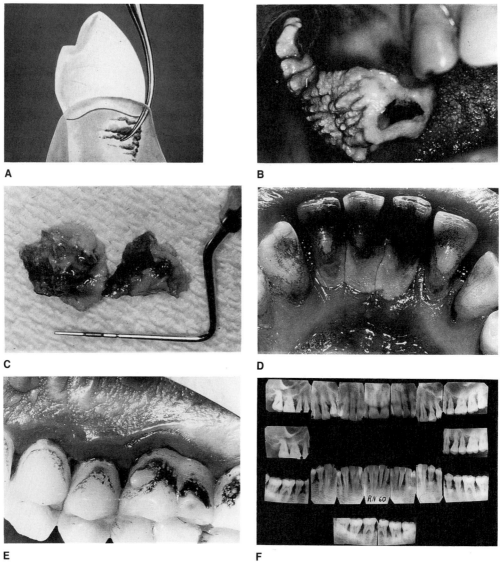

A   **B**

C   **D**

E   **F**

FIGURE 2–22 • Calculus. (*A*) Feeling calculus with an explorer. (Courtesy Dr. TJ O'Leary) (*B*) Supragingival calculus on maxillary molar and premolar area. (*C*) Pieces of calculus measuring approximately 20 mm. (*D*) Large supragingival deposits in mandibular incisor region. (*E*) Subgingival deposits. (*F*) Extensive subgingival calculus is apparent on these radiographs. When obvious etiologic factors like these are present, one can usually expect good results from proper therapy. (*B*) and (*C*) Courtesy of Dr. John Nabers.

Assistant	Doctor
Occlusal Analysis	
	problems wearing complete dentures. Also, tongue thrusters repeatedly compress the uvula and the uvular gag reflex is depressed.
Local Factors	
Bacterial plaque	Note whether plaque stains are present (Fig. 2–21).
Calculus	Note if present and whether supragingival or subgingival (Fig. 2–22).
Interproximal food impaction	Ask patient: "Do meats wedge between your teeth?" Repeat answer to assistant for recording.
Occlusal trauma	Record as present if occlusal analysis showed interfering occlusal contacts or heavy faceting. If these were not found and teeth are not mobile, record as absent.
Blood pressure	Complete oral examination by taking patient's blood pressure. As dentists we see many patients with undiagnosed hypertension. This simple test may be more important to the patient's life than anything else we do.
Mobility	Use instrument handles to exert buccal and lingual pressures on each tooth (Fig. 2–23). It is important that the head be completely immobilized so that only a mobile tooth will move and not the entire head. Immobilization can be achieved either by having your assistant hold the patient's head or by holding the patient's head between your arm and chest. If there is no detectable mobility, do not make any notation on the periodontal chart (see Fig. 2–27). If there is slight mobility that can be perceived visually, record it as first-degree mobility, noted as a *1* in area *a* on the chart. If there is mobility of 1 mm or more buccal–lingually, record it as a *2*. If tooth shows excessive buccal–lingual movement and can be depressed in the socket by apical pressure with an instrument handle, record it as a *3*. Record all teeth with class 3 mobility that are to be retained as having a guarded long-term prognosis and formulate the restorative treatment plan accordingly.

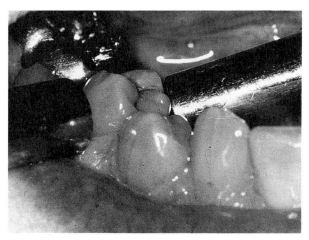

FIGURE **2–23** • Testing mobility by exerting pressure on the tooth with an instrument handle.

Assistant	Doctor
Local Factors	
Open contacts	Use thin unwaxed floss to test contacts between all teeth (Fig. 2–24). If floss goes through easily and no restorations are present, put a *1* in area *b* on chart beneath appropriate tooth (see Fig. 2–27). If you find an open contact with floss that requires restoration, record it as a 2. If patient has detected food impaction in area, circle number that you place on chart. This notation means that if open contact and food impaction persists after corrective periodontal therapy, restorative procedures are required to establish good bracing contact (Fig. 2–25).
Vitality	Test vitality of tooth with electric vitalometer and record reading with numerical grade at location *c* under appropriate tooth (see Fig. 2–27).
Pocket probing	Six surfaces are probed on each tooth and depth is recorded in millimeters. These surfaces are as follows (see Fig. 2–27):

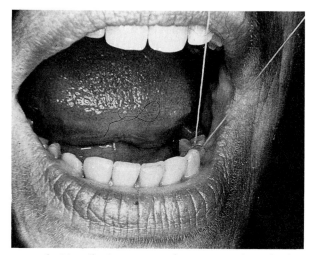

FIGURE **2–24** • Testing contact between teeth with thin unwaxed floss.

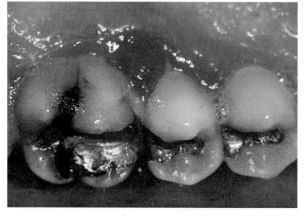

FIGURE **2–25** • Contact between teeth. Inflamed interproximal tissue is apparent in area where contact was totally open. Patient had been packing food in the area chronically. Treatment was replacement of both restorations.

Assistant	Doctor
Local Factors	

<table>
<tr><td></td><td>d, distobuccal   g, distolingual
e, buccal   h, lingual
f, mesiobuccal   i, mesiolingual</td></tr>
</table>

To determine amount of probing force to be used, place end of probe on your fingertip and press until blanching just starts to occur. This will give you a good estimate of force to be used. Before probing, explain to the patient that you are going to see how far this diagnostic instrument goes under the gums and that 1 or 2 mm is ideal. Explain that depths beyond 3 mm are called "pockets" and that these harbor bacteria and produce pus. Explain that as the pocket goes deeper, bone will be destroyed. When pockets are present around old restorations, check margins for discrepancies that hold bacterial plaque. If probing pocket depth is very painful discontinue probing and explain that you will probe only a few teeth. The x-ray films usually reveal areas where depth of bone destruction is greatest, and those areas need to be probed. In patients with extreme sensitivity, subgingival scaling procedures are performed using a local anesthetic. When such scaling procedures are performed later, complete probing can be done at the same time.

Furcation probing

Using furcation probes (Fig. 2–26), probe furcation areas to see if there is involvement or not. One of the main reasons to determine furcation involvement by probing is to better determine prognosis of multirooted involved teeth. This has great bearing on restorative treatment planning. Record all teeth with Class II or Class III furcation involvement with a question mark to indicate doubtful prognosis. The final restorative treatment plan must be formulated with the realization that these teeth may be lost later. Furcation involvements are indicated as follows:

A starting or Class I furcation is recorded with one bar across the line (Fig. 2–27, *j*).

A Class II involvement has started into the furcation, but is not in all the way (Fig. 2–27, *k*).

A Class III trifurcation involvement is one that is in all the way from the buccal and the distal (Fig. 2–27, *l*).

Class I, Class II, and Class III bifurcation involvements found by the furcation probing are shown as *m, n,* and *o* in Figure 2–27. A straight probe will not usually detect a furcation involvement.

Other notations that can be recorded on the chart are as follows:

p: A line that depicts the mucogingival junction (also called a flap line).

q: A recording of a pocket that is apical to the mucogingival junction where it would be necessary to do a flap procedure rather than a gingivoplasty. (A gingivoplasty incision should never be within alveolar mucosa.)

r: A diagonal line across the tooth indicates this tooth is to be extracted.

s: The X and the blackened-out occlusal part indicate a missing tooth.

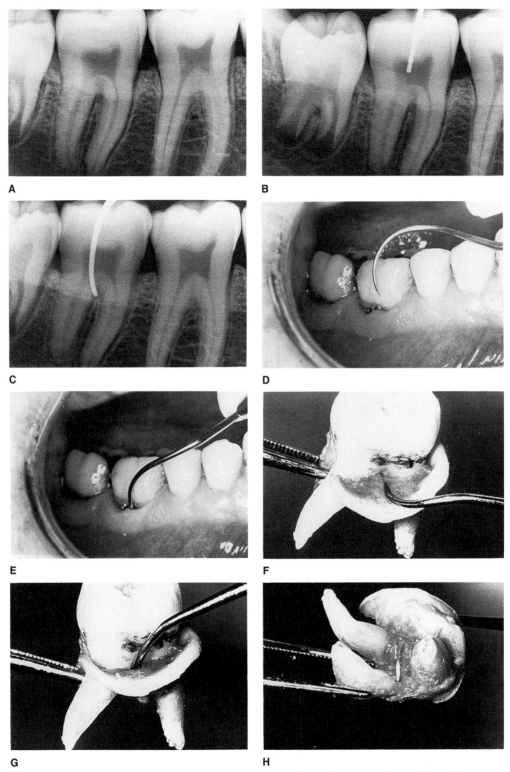

FIGURE 2–26 ● Furcation probing. (*A*) Radiograph of molars. The widened periodontal ligaments visible here indicate the presence of occlusal trauma. (*B*) Probing the furcation with a straight probe. (*C*) Probing the furcation with a special curved probe. (*D*) Special probe to determine furcation involvement. (*E*) Probe going into furcation area. (*F*) Furcation probe to be used on an extracted tooth with retained gingival tissues. (*G*) Probe in place. (*H*) View of the furcation with the probe in place. (*F–H*, Courtesy Dr. Bobby Romans)

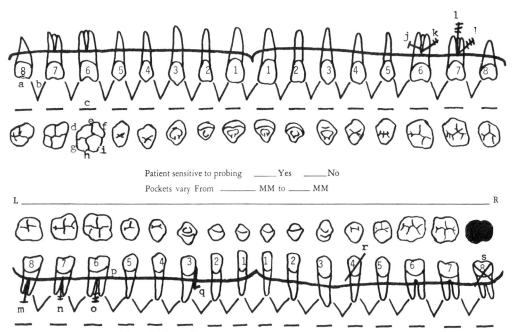

FIGURE 2–27 • A periodontal chart showing notations to document various clinical conditions (see text for descriptions).

Diagnostic Tests

In summary, the diagnostic procedures used in the initial periodontal assessment are as follows:

Clinical intra- and extraoral examination
Radiographic examination
Occlusal examination
Tests of tooth mobility
Tests of tooth vitality
Periodontal examination

In addition, if necessary, a biopsy may also need to be performed. The clinician should also measure the blood glucose with a glucometer if there is any reason to suspect that patient may be diabetic.

When the diagnostic procedures are completed, the patient will know that you have a thorough understanding of what you are doing and of the problems present. At this time you should explain that these tests are needed to identify what problems are present so that you can determine what corrective procedures are required. Your objective is to do the minimum that is needed in order to obtain the best and most maintainable result so that the patient can keep his teeth in good health. (Be sure that the patient understands that you plan to follow this principle of treatment.)

Biopsy

Biopsy is often required during periodontal therapy. The patient must be informed both of the need for biopsy and, when they become available, of the results.

INDICATIONS

Biopsy is indicated in the following circumstances:
1. When you cannot make a clinical diagnosis without it.
2. To confirm your clinical diagnosis.
3. When cancer is a remote possibility. If you think cancer is a probable diagnosis, refer the patient to a doctor or a clinic that normally treats cancer.

OBJECTIVE

The acquisition of a tissue sample for microscopic examination for the purpose of establishing a diagnosis is the objective. The biopsy is sometimes needed for the patient's peace of mind as well as for medicolegal documentation.

TECHNIQUES

1. When possible, ensure that the section removed contains healthy tissue as well as tissue from the area of interest. Always remove the entire lesion when possible (Fig. 2–28).
2. Orient the section for the pathologist by placing a tail on the distal side so that the sections can be properly cut.

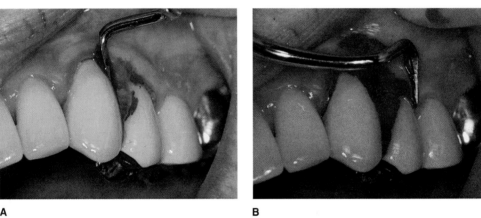

A   B

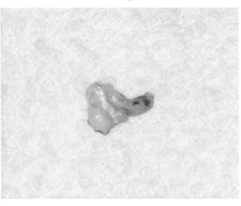

C

FIGURE 2–28 • Biopsy technique. (A) Incising a hyperplastic inflamed papilla mesial to the maxillary first premolar crown. The lesion had not healed despite several therapies by the patient's general dentist. (B) A tail of healthy tissue is included on the distal aspect in order to orient the specimen for the pathologist. (C) The removed papilla with distal tail after washing in water and before placing in a fixing solution. The pathologist reported chronic inflammation. This was caused by rough crown margins, which were smoothed during the biopsy procedure.

3. Place the biopsy sample in a fixing solution after rinsing the blood off with water.
4. Send a detailed description and history with the sample so that the pathologist will have as much information as possible when making the diagnosis.
5. Ensure that x-ray films accompany the biopsy when pertinent.

Grafting may be necessary to restore normal anatomy (Figs. 2–29, 2–30).

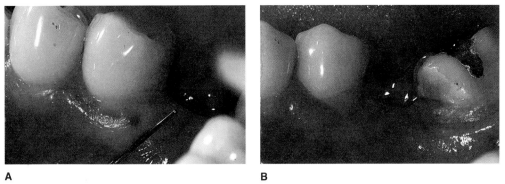

A   **B**

FIGURE 2–29 • Biopsy and grafting. (A) Blanching with probe before biopsy shows lesion is not inflammatory in nature, since it does not disappear. The lesion was excised and a free gingival graft was used for repair. The pathology report showed that the lesion was a cavernous hemangioma. (B) Appearance 1 month after biopsy and repair.

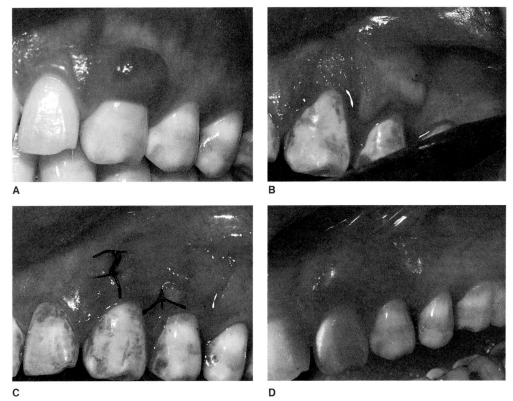

A   **B**

C   **D**

FIGURE 2–30 • Biopsy and grafting. (A) Lesion on the facial aspect of the maxillary canine. The lesion had been present for 1 year and was treated twice with curettage, under assumption that it was an abscess. This treatment proved ineffective, so patient was referred for periodontal diagnosis and treatment. (B) Excisional biopsy was performed. (C) A tissue pedicle was moved from the distal side to replace the gingiva. (D) Appearance 1 week after surgery. Histologic diagnosis was pyogenic granuloma. The lesion healed uneventfully and normal periodontal architecture was restored.

Sequential Treatment Plan

As already mentioned, the objective of periodontal therapy is to achieve the best and most maintainable result possible, while doing no more work than is necessary. Use the following sequential treatment plan outline as a check list, starting at the top and working down, skipping any steps that are not indicated. All these procedures are covered in detail in subsequent chapters.

INITIAL PREPARATION

Medical consultation and treatment.
Suggested dietary changes and/or prescribed supplements.
Control of deep caries and endodontic therapy.
Extraction of hopelessly involved teeth with temporary replacements where needed.
Scalings and removal of overhanging margins—may require local anesthesia.
Instructions on personal oral hygiene and physiotherapy.
Instructions for patients needing change in parafunction occlusal habits.
Reexamination, reevaluation after six-week interval. Decisions to proceed with corrective therapy should be based on the patient's home care and response to initial therapy as well as problems that are still present.
Subgingival curettage with local anesthesia, reinstruction on oral hygiene, and review of dietary habits, occlusal habits, etc.
Occlusal adjustments and planning for needed corrective therapy.
Orthodontic treatment for minor tooth movement.
Temporary or provisional splinting for severe periodontitis when required to stabilize mobile teeth with secondary occlusal traumatism.

CORRECTIVE THERAPY

Periodontal surgery, including resective and regenerative procedures.
Correction of mucogingival problems and treatment of multirooted teeth with root amputations and hemisections.
Postsurgical treatment of hypersensitive teeth.
A minimum 3-month wait following extensive periodontal surgery prior to restorative dentistry, fixed bridges, fixed splinting, partial dentures, etc. This interval will allow connective tissue attachments to the teeth to mature and heal.
Occlusal rechecks with refinements of occlusion and adjustments of mitigatory occlusal habit appliances. This is necessary because of rebounding of mobile teeth and minor changes of tooth positions.

MAINTENANCE AND CORRECTIVE FOLLOW-UP CARE

Assessment of patient's oral hygiene efficiency.
Scaling, root planing, subgingival curettage where indicated, and probing of each surface of each tooth every 3 to 6 months. Mobility of the teeth should be tested and the entire mouth should be examined and checked for visible caries.

Completion of x-ray coverage when dictated by patient's disease activity and periodic comparison with prior x-rays.

Removal, checking, and recementing, every 1 to 2 years, of any fixed splints that are temporarily cemented. This should be done by the doctor who made the splint. When it is apparent the patient is having no problems, permanent cementation should be considered.

Treatment of any new pockets that develop.

Treatment of any new caries that develop.

Endodontic therapy, if indicated.

Replacement of restorations or bridges that no longer satisfy esthetic, functional, or health requirements.

Creation of new mitigatory occlusal habit appliances when old ones are broken down, worn out, or lost.

For drop-out patients returning in real trouble or patients with unexplainable serious problems, initial preparation or corrective therapy or referral to someone else.

Sample Treatment Plan

Several different treatment plans will now be discussed, starting with the simplest case possible and proceeding to more difficult cases. Since most private practitioners deal heavily with third-party-payment plans, the appropriate insurance code number is included in each treatment plan. The significance of these numbers is as follows:

04500	Gingivitis: shallow pockets, no bone loss.
04600	Early periodontitis: moderate pockets, minor-to-moderate bone loss, satisfactory topography.
04700	Moderate periodontitis: moderate-to-deep pockets, moderate-to-severe bone loss, unsatisfactory topography.
04800	Advanced periodontitis: deep pockets, severe bone loss, advanced mobility patterns (usually missing teeth and reconstruction cases).
04900	Refractory progressive periodontitis: periodontitis which does not respond to conventional therapy.

For treatment purposes, these categories can be further subdivided as outlined in the following sections.

SIMPLE MARGINAL GINGIVITIS WITH NO POCKETS AND NO CALCULUS (04500)

Schedule the patient for four weekly 30-minute appointments, during which the preventive nurse should instruct him on effective plaque control and gingival physiotherapy. At each of these appointments ask the patient to wash his hands and demonstrate his oral hygiene techniques. Minor corrections are always needed, but only point these out after complimenting the patient. After the first appointment, instruct the patient to floss and brush an hour before these appointments. Start each visit by using a plaque stain; the nurse can then show the patient where he has missed. At the end of each of these treatments, all the teeth should be polished with a rubber cup using commercial polishing material. A high shine on the teeth helps the patient with plaque control. Always floss the polishing material from the interproximals afterwards.

GINGIVITIS WITH SUPRAGINGIVAL AND SUBGINGIVAL CALCULUS, BUT NO EVIDENCE OF BONE LOSS AND INTACT GINGIVAL PAPILLAE WHEN POCKET DEPTH DOES NOT EXCEED 3 MM (04500)

Follow the same routine as in the preceding case, but add 1 hour at the first and third appointments for thorough scaling of the teeth. Root planing is indicated if there is exudate or detectable subgingival accretions on the roots.

GINGIVITIS WITH CALCIFIED DEPOSITS AND MINOR BONE LOSS BUT WITH POOR GINGIVAL CONTOURS OR BROKEN PAPILLAE AND POCKET DEPTH OF 3 TO 5 MM DUE TO GINGIVAL ENLARGEMENT (04600)

Follow the same routine as in the preceding case, but plan to reappoint the patient for 6 weeks later to reevaluate the possible need for surgical correction of any still-existing deviations from normal. The patient must understand the specific fee up to this point and that the fee for any needed surgical corrective treatment will be determined at reevaluation.

PERIODONTITIS WITH SLIGHT BONE LOSS AND WITH HIGHLY INFLAMMED GINGIVAE (04600)

Follow the same procedure as in the preceding case.

CHRONIC PERIODONTITIS WITH SLIGHT BONE LOSS AND WITH FIBROUS GINGIVAL HYPERPLASIA (04600)

Follow the same procedures as in the preceding case, but plan from the beginning that surgery will be needed after the initial preparation. The treatment plan for the surgical phase of treatment follows:

Make the patient's appointment for 30 minutes before the time reserved for you so that the patient can be premedicated if necessary. Be sure the patient has a responsible adult to take him home. About 1½ to 2 hours will be needed to operate on the right or left side of the mouth when a full complement of teeth is present. Prescribe systemic antibiotics when indicated (see Table 2–1).

Table 2–1 • INDICATIONS FOR SYSTEMIC ANTIBIOTIC COVERAGE

Congenital heart disease
  Ventricular septal defect
  Tetralogy of Fallot
  Aortic stenosis
  Pulmonary stenosis
  Complex cyanotic heart disease
  Patient ductus arteriosus
  Systemic to pulmonary artery shunts
Rheumatic heart disease or other acquired valvular heart disease
Idiopathic hypertrophic subaortic stenosis
Mitral valve prolapse
Prosthetic heart valves
Diabetes mellitus
Joint prosthesis: Hip/knee
Renal transplant or dialysis
Also consider antibiotics for patients who have undergone
  Pacemaker insertion
  Irradiation to head and neck
  Coronary by-pass procedures
  Osseous grafting procedures
(Courtesy Dr. Steven Bricker)

After the last dressing is removed, make three appointments at 2-week intervals for the preventive nurse to recheck flossing and brushing and for the teeth to be polished by rubber cupping with a high-shine polishing agent.

On the last appointment scale, polish, and check the results, and with a mirror show the patient the end result (no pockets, no inflammation, and contours that can be maintained). If preoperative photographs were taken, be sure to photograph the end results.

PERIODONTITIS WITH MODERATE-TO-SEVERE BONE LOSS IN WHICH POCKETS HAVE PROGRESSED TO THE POINT WHERE OSSEOUS DEFECTS REQUIRING OSSEOUS SURGERY ARE PRESENT (04800)

Follow the same procedures as in the preceding case, but allocate about 1½ to 2 hours for each quadrant. The extra time is required when osseous surgery is performed not only because flaps must be incised and sutured in the proper positions, but also because special care is needed in dressing placement. Osseous surgery may include bone fill, osseous contouring, autogenous bone graft, apical repositioning of a gingival graft flap, or tissue-guided regeneration.

REFRACTORY PROGRESSIVE PERIODONTITIS (04900)

Refractory progressive periodontitis includes several unclassified types of periodontitis characterized by either rapid or continuous bone and attachment loss.

These rare diseases do not respond to normal therapy. Patients with these diseases should be referred, since they will frequently require microbiologic and antibody evaluation, followed by combined mechanical and chemotherapeutic treatment. Consult with your dental school about referrals if you have not yet developed a working relationship with a periodontist.

Microbiological Etiology of Periodontal Diseases*

Prior to 1965, there were several divergent views of the primary cause of periodontal disease. In 1965, Harald Löe demonstrated very clearly that gingival inflammation was caused solely by the increase in bacterial plaque accumulations on the teeth. From this observation many studies followed which associated plaque accumulations with not only gingivitis but also periodontitis. Other studies demonstrated that plaque removal was very effective in both preventing and treating periodontal diseases. What emerged from these studies was a theory that the amount of plaque determined the initiation and progression of periodontal disease. This concept was extended by some to the conclusion that the amount of plaque was the only thing that mattered in the development of periodontal disease.

Beginning in the mid 1970s, with the development of new technologies, it became possible to take a more extensive look at the roles of the host and specific bacteria in the periodontal disease process. This work was instigated to a great extent by the clinical observations of astute practitioners. Many noticed that some patients failed to respond predictably to the best conventional periodontal care available in spite of good home care and good professional maintenance. It was also clear that in some cases the extent of destruction could not be related to the amount of plaque, the age of the patient, or the duration of exposure to plaque.

Today it appears that there are several different forms of periodontal disease, most likely involving different bacteria as well as in some cases different immunologic and inflammatory responses. Although the terminology is not uniform, there is a general acceptance that several distinct forms of periodontal disease exist. It should be emphasized that we know very little about the long-term response to treatment of these forms of periodontal disease. Current classification systems will be of only academic interest unless different diseases can be shown to respond differently to therapy. At present it is important to attempt to separate the different clinical presentations of disease in order to monitor and catalog responses to therapy.

Several distinct clinical forms of periodontal disease can now be recognized. The disease which we know the most about, in terms of therapeutic response, might be termed "Adult Periodontitis." This is the disease that we most commonly see in our patients. It generally is first detected after the age of 35 and is associated with moderate to heavy accumulations of plaque and calculus. Gingivitis is clearly evident and the radiographic evidence of bone loss generally demonstrates a horizontal pattern, although localized defects may be present. Adult periodontitis has

---

*Contributed by Dr. Kenneth Kornman, Chairman of the Department of Periodontics, University of Texas Health Science Center, San Antonio, Texas.

been associated with several bacteria. Some of the most common are *Bacteroides gingivalis, Bacteroides intermedius,* and other *Bacteroides* species, spirochetes, *Fusobacterium* species, *Eubacterium* species, and *Wolinella recta.* Adult periodontitis may turn out to have the most complex microbial pattern of all periodontal diseases, since one is faced with individualized host–parasite interactions in different patients.

Another group of diseases may be classified as "early-onset periodontitis." This category includes localized juvenile periodontitis, prepubertal periodontitis, and some forms of rapidly progressive periodontitis. Localized juvenile periodontitis is thought to occur sometime after puberty and is detectable before the age of 20. The disease is localized to the first molars and (often) the incisors, and is generally associated with minimal clinical levels of plaque and calculus. These patients are known to have a defect in white blood cell function and a unique microbial plaque that includes *Actinobacillus actinomycetemcomitans.* Prepubertal periodontitis is thought to begin before puberty, is seen in the primary dentition, and may be either generalized to most of the dentition or localized to just a few teeth. This disease is also associated with a defect in either neutrophil or monocyte function. Preliminary reports indicate that these patients are colonized early by the potential periodontal pathogens *Actinobacillus actinomycetemcomitans, Bacteroides intermedius, Capnocytophaga sputigena,* and *Eikenella corrodens.* Generalized severe destruction of the peridontium may also be seen in postpubertal adolescents. This presentation has been termed generalized juvenile periodontitis or, by some, rapidly progressive periodontitis. In some of these cases, the disease clearly originates as a localized juvenile periodontitis and spreads to other teeth, but it is not yet clear whether this reflects distinct entities or different presentations of a single disease. Likewise, the microbiology of such conditions is not well defined.

Another clinical presentation is severe periodontal disease with variable local factors in an individual over the age of 35. Usually as practitioners we do not have the luxury of knowing the history of such cases. Since these cases generally appear different from adult periodontitis either in terms of severity of bone loss and loss of attachment, or in terms of minimal local factors, it seems appropriate to separate them into a distinct classification. At present the most common terminology for such cases is rapidly progressive periodontitis. This name, of course, suggests that the disease occurs "rapidly" during a given period, even though such longitudinal observations may not be possible. In practice, these cases usually present as disease that seems exceptionally severe in relation to the accompanying local factors. Every practitioner with a well-established maintenance practice also has within his practice a certain percentage of cases which present recurrent problems. These have been categorized as "Refractory Periodontitis" in an effort to indicate that they do not respond predictably to conventional periodontal therapy. Although little is known about them, preliminary studies in such cases indicate that a specific small group of bacteria can routinely be isolated from the sites of progressive diseases.

There are several other conditions that should be noted either because they are newly recognized entities or because we have gained additional knowledge about their etiology. We now know that pregnancy-associated gingivitis, pregnancy-associated periodontitis, and acute necrotizing ulcerative gingivitis are associated with elevated levels of *Bacteroides intermedius.* This bacterium appears to increase during systemic changes in hormonal levels, such as those that accompany pregnancy or stress.

Two newly recognized conditions are HIV periodontitis and HIV gingivitis. As the names suggest, these diseases are associated with HIV infections. HIV periodontitis may present as an acute necrotizing ulcerative gingivitis with associated episodes of rapid bone loss and loss of attachment. HIV gingivitis generally presents as a well-defined generalized gingivitis at the marginal gingiva which is not predictably responsive to local therapy. Preliminary studies indicate that HIV periodontal diseases are associated with elevated levels of *Bacteroides intermedius, Wolinella recta,* and certain other gram-negative surface-translocating bacteria (Fig. 2–31).

As noted above, these diseases appear to be distinct clinical, microbiological, and immunologic entities. Although several studies have indicated that localized juvenile periodontitis does not respond predictably to conventional periodontal therapy, few data are available on the other conditions. Future work in this area must determine specific means of diagnosing each condition and document the long-term response to various therapies.

Bibliography

Current Procedural Terminology for Periodontics. 5th edition. American Academy of Periodontology, 1986.

DeVore CH, et al. Retained "hopeless" teeth: Effects on the proximal periodontium of adjacent teeth. J Periodontol 1988; 59:647–651.

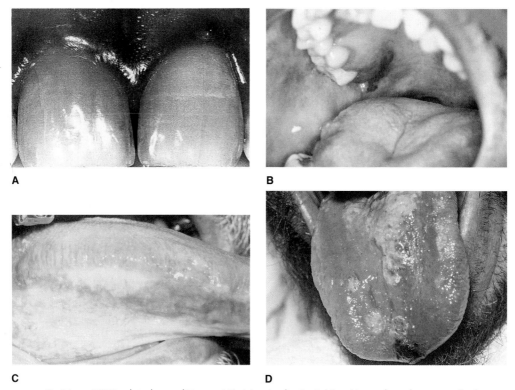

A   B

C   D

FIGURE **2–31** • AIDS-related conditions. (*A*) Marginal gingivitis. Note the absence of plaque. (*B*) Kaposi's sarcoma lesion in hard palate. (*C*) Hairy leukoplakia, right lateral border. (*D*) Multiple lesions on dorsum of tongue secondary to reactivation of herpes simplex virus. (*A*, Courtesy Dr. Ken Kornman; *B–D*, Courtesy Dr. Spencer Redding)

Ebersole JL, et al. Human serum antibody responses to oral microorganisms IV. Correlation with homologous infection. Oral Microbiol Immunol 1987; 2:53–59.

Garliner D. Myofunctional therapy in dental practice. 2nd ed. Brooklyn: Bartel Dental Book Company, 1974.

Goldman HM, Stallard RE. Limitations of the radiograph in the diagnosis of osseous defects in periodontal disease. J Periodontol 1973; 44:626–628.

Keagle JG, et al. Gingival resistance to probing forces. I. Determination of optimal probe diameter. J Periodontol 1989; 60:167–171.

Keszthelyi G, Szabo I. Influence of class II amalgam fillings on attachment loss. J Clin Periodontol 1984; 11(2):81–86.

Kornman KS, Loesche WJ. The subgingival microbial flora during pregnancy. J Clin Periodont 1980; 15(2):111–122.

Kramer GM. A consideration of root proximity. Int J Periodont Res Dent 1987; V(6):9–34.

Lang NP, et al. Clinical and microbiological effects of subgingival restorations with overhanging or clinically perfect margins. J Clin Periodontol 1983; 10:563–578.

Listgarten MA, Mao R, Robinson PJ. Periodontal probing and the relationship of the probe tip to periodontal tissues. J Periodontol 1976; 47:511–513.

Proceedings from the State of the Art Workshop on Surgical Therapy for Periodontitis. J Periodontol 1982; 53:475–501.

Ramfjord SP, et al. Longitudinal study of periodontal therapy. J Periodontol 1973; 44:66–77.

Tanner ACR, Socransky SS, Goodson JM. Microbiota of periodontal pockets losing crestal alveolar bone. J Periodont Res 1984; 19:279–291.

Warner DA, Sims TN. Periodontal probing: A review. J West Soc Periodontol 1982; 30:132–138.

CHAPTER THREE

Emergency Procedures

Emergency dental care is one of the most important services a dentist provides. It not only relieves pain and suffering but exposes many patients to modern dentistry for the first time. The primary goal of emergency periodontal treatment should be the elimination of pain. X-rays, periodontal and dental diagnosis, and treatment planning should follow elimination of pain.

The Periodontal Abscess

The first objective in treating the abscess is to establish drainage. This should relieve the pain and start resolution of the infection. Antibiotics may be used if the abscess is spreading into adjacent anatomic spaces, if the patient is feeling bad as a result of the infection or is running a fever or, especially, if the abscess is in an area of the mouth, such as the anterior maxilla, where spreading of the infection could have dire consequences. Drainage may be established through the sulcus, or by incision and drainage (lancing) if the abscess has pointed (Fig. 3–1). Patients will frequently recall eating popcorn 2 or 3 days before the abscess developed, and a popcorn husk will often be found when the abscess is incised.

Establishment of drainage through the sulcus is more challenging clinically because locating the base of the abscess may be more difficult. Use a thin probe with gentle pressure, going firmly and thoroughly around the sulcus until the probe drops into the lesion. Widen the opening with small files or curettes until pus begins to exude (Fig. 3–2).

After the acute phase has subsided a chronic inflammatory lesion will often remain. A resulting pocket should be treated thoroughly, usually with a full-thickness flap for access, as soon as possible after the acute phase is over. This is done to minimize attachment loss and maximize the repair potential of the bone.

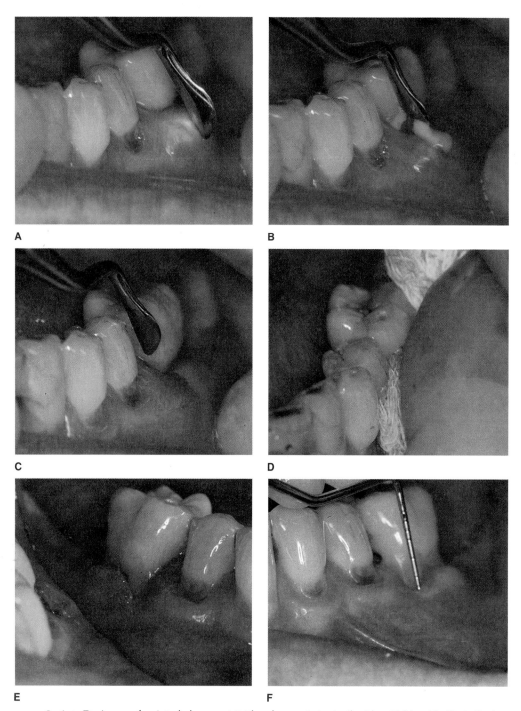

A

B

C

D

E

F

FIGURE **3–1** • Drainage of pointed abscess. (*A*) The abscess is incised with a Kirkland knife 15K after a mandibular and long buccal anesthetic has been given. (*B*) The incision is made to the bone. Suppurative exudate flows from abscess. (*C*) The area is squeezed from all directions toward the incision to squeeze the pus out. (*D*) After thorough irrigation of the abscess area with sterile normal saline, gauze is used to compress the tissues of the tooth. Moderate pressure for 3 minutes helps form a thin fibrin clot to glue the tissues in place. (*E*) A mirror view of the area after the gauze is removed. (*F*) Area of abscess being probed 8 weeks later. The probe depth is only 1.5 mm, showing that no residual pocket is present.

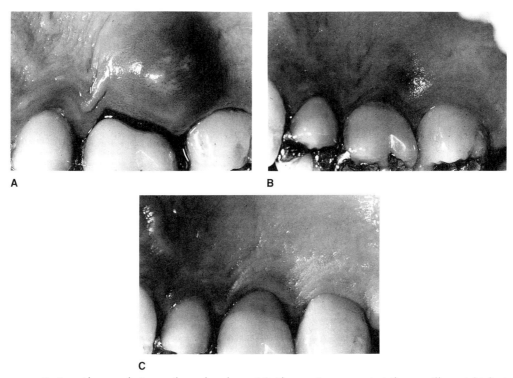

FIGURE 3–2 • Abscess drainage through sulcus. (*A*) Abscess is apparent at the maxillary right first molar on lingual aspect in a patient seen on an emergency appointment. (*B*) Same area 2 weeks later. Drainage was established through the sulcus. No incision was made. (*C*) Same area 3 months after pocket elimination surgery.

Acute Necrotizing Ulcerative Gingivitis

This acute and often painful disease can be vexing. Most patients suffering from acute necrotizing ulcerative gingivitis are under emotional stress, such as final examinations in school, marital disharmony, or financial strain, or are physically debilitated. They are sometimes unreliable patients who do not pay their dental bills and stop treatments when the acute stage has been resolved and the pain is eliminated. If this happens, the patient may lose his teeth later in life. The following are aids to treating these patients effectively and thoroughly: Have the patient who can, pay for full-mouth x-rays and for 2 hours of therapy before starting treatment. Explain to the patient that after completing this contracted initial treatment to get him (or her) out of pain, you will be in a position to tell him what else will be needed. If the patient has a temperature over 100° F and/or lymphadenopathy of the submaxillary, submental, or cervical lymph nodes, place him on a systemic antibiotic. Have the patient floss with unwaxed floss and apply chlorhexidine mouth wash to his toothbrush, then brush only the teeth and not the gums. This should be done after breakfast, after lunch, and before going to bed as his home treatment. After each flossing and brushing home care treatment, the patient should swish vigorously for 2 full minutes with chlorhexidine mouth rinse. When the acute phase is over, discontinue the use of chlorhexidine. Plan on four half-hour

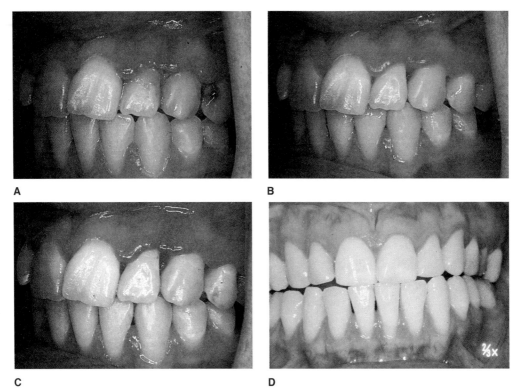

FIGURE 3–3 • Acute necrotizing ulcerative gingivitis. (*A*) Left side of patient seen on emergency for gingival pain. A topical anesthetic was given, the necrotic material was debrided, and the pockets were scaled out. (*B*) Left side 2 days after debridement. Patient stated she felt much better. (*C*) Left side 6 weeks later. The pain and inflammation were gone, but gingival deformities were still apparent. (*D*) Appearance 26 years after gingivoplasty to correct deformities.

appointments. Start by removing all necrotic ulcerative materials and scale out the pockets to remove calculus and to establish vascular and lymphatic drainage (Fig. 3–3 A,B). A topical anesthetic may be necessary for the first treatment as there is active hyperemia in the tissues, and the nerves are hypersensitive. In only a few minutes of instrumentation, the pain will decrease about 50% because of the decrease in pressure within the tissues. Our experience has been that if treated early and thoroughly, and there had been no previous occurrences, the punched-out interdental papillae regenerate completely (Fig. 3-3 C,D).

Herpes Simplex Gingivostomatitis

A painful viral infection, herpes simplex gingivostomatitis may follow dental appointments (Fig. 3–4), toothbrush trauma, floss cuts (Fig. 3–5), high fever, colds, or gastrointestinal upsets. It can occur on the lips as well as in the mouth. Patients cannot and will not maintain good oral hygiene while in pain—which usually lasts only about 7 days. It is important to distinguish this infection from other inflammatory gingival lesions such as bacterial and allergic reactions because treatment must be guided by the diagnosis. Palliative treatment is helpful and will be discussed in the section on primary herpetic gingivostomatitis. To avoid contracting a herpetic lesion, always use rubber gloves when examining any patient.

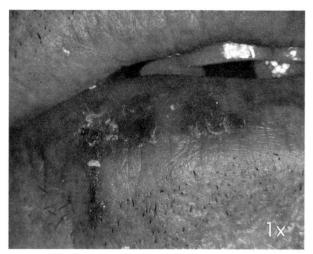

FIGURE 3–4 • Recurring herpes simplex on the lip after dental treatment.

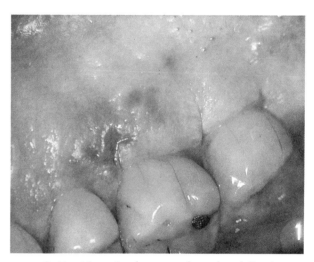

FIGURE 3–5 • Herpetic cluster on the palate following repeated floss cutting.

Primary Herpetic Gingivostomatitis

Primary herpetic gingivostomatitis is probably the most painful gingival disease. It is most frequently seen in children 2 to 5 years old (Fig. 3–6). The older the adult patient with primary herpes, the more painful and severe is the disease (Figs. 3–7, 3–8). There is no known cure. When primary herpetic gingivostomatitis occurs, for the patient's peace of mind and to rule out blood dyscrasias, and so on, have his physician do blood chemistries and a complete blood count. Expect the temperature to possibly go up to 104° F within 2 days after onset. An important factor in making this diagnosis is that the patient has never had a fever blister (herpes simplex) in his lifetime, and therefore has no antibodies or resistance. Wear rubber

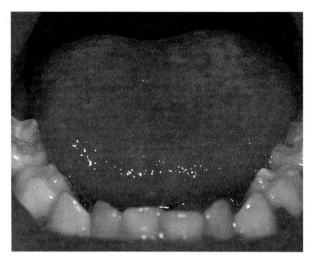

FIGURE **3–6** • Primary herpes on tongue of a 2-year-old male.

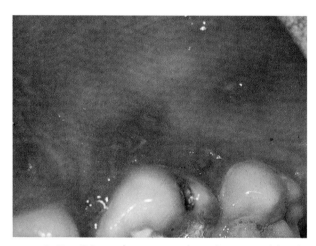

FIGURE **3–7** • Primary herpes on palate of 20-year-old male 4 days after onset.

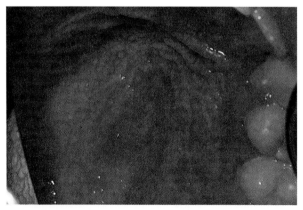

FIGURE **3–8** • Primary herpes on palate of another 20-year-old male 8 days after onset. Lesions have coalesced, making it more difficult to distinguish them from other vesiculo-ulcerative lesions.

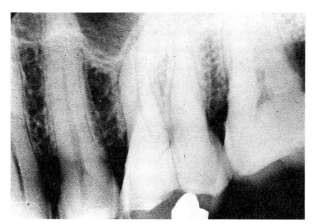

FIGURE 3–9 • Radiograph of a tooth with a fracture. (This is seldom detectable on x-ray images.)

gloves to examine this patient (and all others). The duration of the high fever and general malaise is approximately 7 to 9 days. Antibiotics are indicated only in cases of secondary infection. Instruct the patient to avoid highly seasoned food and to avoid contact with gingival tissues when brushing and flossing. Chlorhexidine rinses are very helpful in controlling plaque during the acute phase. A treatment for palliative relief is:*

Elixir of Dimetapp   100 cc
Kaopectate   200 cc
Distilled water   300 cc
Sig.: Rinse as often as needed for temporary relief of pain. Expecto-
      rate after rinsing for 1/2 minute. Do not swallow.

Some patients with this rare viral infection need to be hospitalized to control temperature. In 50 years of practice, we have seen 6 adults suffering from this infection.

Cracked Tooth Syndrome

Until 20 years ago, the diagnosis and treatment of a cracked tooth presented a most exasperating emergency problem. Unless the tooth could be seen to be fractured, the workup consisted of studying x-ray films, testing vitality, adjusting occlusion, and percussing teeth. These tests were all nondiagnostic (Fig. 3–9). Since then, the use of the anesthetic carpule rubber stopper with floss threaded through it (or the equivalent use of a thick rubber band) has made diagnosis easier and more accurate (Fig. 3–10). If the cracked tooth is vital, prepare it for a temporary crown, making sure all cusps are completely covered. If the tooth becomes asymptomatic and is still vital 4 to 6 weeks later, make a permanent crown for it. We have found that diagonal fractures involving the pulp and extending to the mid root or apical third of the root require extraction, since endodontic therapy, and crowns will not be effective in over 95% of such cases (Fig. 3–11).

*Developed by Dr. William C. Hurt

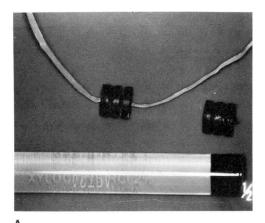
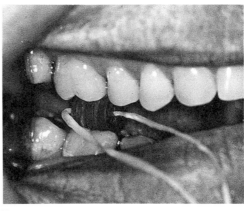

A   **B**

FIGURE **3–10** • Detection of a cracked tooth. (A) One plunge is removed from a dental anesthetic carpule and floss is threaded through another. (B) The patient bites on rubber stopper. If he has a cracked tooth, biting and opening will usually cause the cracked pieces to open or come back together, causing pain.

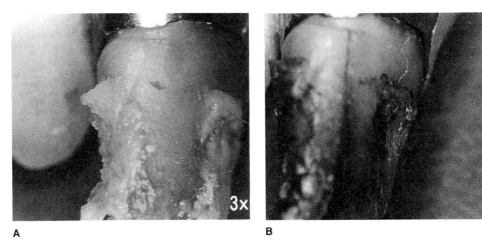

A   **B**

FIGURE **3–11** • Cracked tooth syndrome. (A) This extracted tooth had been causing extreme pain for 3 weeks. No crack was evident, but one was suspected because a deep, rapidly developing pocket was present. (B) The cracked tooth was dried and covered with methylene blue. After rinsing the vertical fracture which was the cause of pain is revealed.

Retrograde Periodontitis

Infrequently, periodontal or pulpal pathosis creates a combined pulpal-periodontal lesion. Treatment is described later. The first challenge is diagnosis. Always suspect pulpal involvement if the patient on emergency appointment responds in answer to questioning that hot hurts and cold feels good or that the pain is a throbbing pain. Vitality testing, percussion, and periapical x-ray studies aid in determining pulpal involvement. When there is a chronic sinus tract with drainage of purulent material

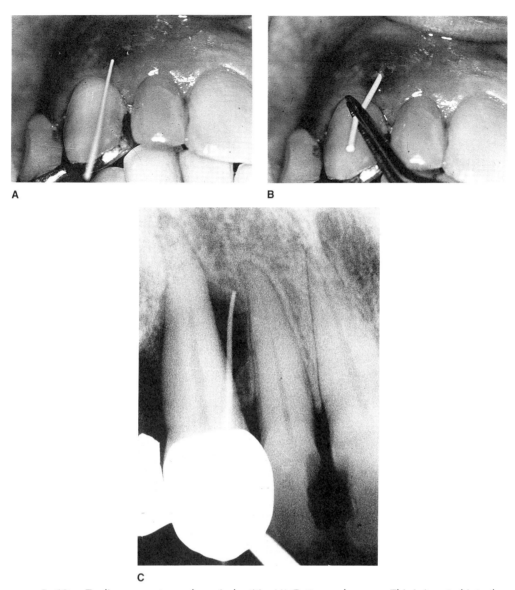

A

B

C

FIGURE 3–12 • To diagnose retrograde periodontitis. (*A*) Gutta percha cone. This is inserted into the area of the abscess. (*B*) Gutta percha cone placed to bottom of abscess before x-ray. (*C*) X-ray film showing the source of infection. This shows that the source of infection was not from the apex.

out of a raised lump, it is highly likely that the pulp is involved. One aid in diagnosis is to place a gutta-percha point into the fistulous tract and push it in as far as possible until it is stopped by a resistant tissue (Fig. 3–12 A,B). Then x-ray the area to see where the point of the gutta percha is (Fig. 3–12 C). The gutta percha probe will stop at the apex of the pulpally involved tooth. If there is no pulpal pathosis the end of the probe will be away from the apex. To test vitality on crowned teeth, it may be necessary to drill a hole through the crown and bur into the dentin. Keep in mind that collateral canals can occur in areas of furcations, so all teeth with furcation involvements should be checked for pulpal pathosis. Endodontic therapy or extraction are the possible solutions to the pulpal pathosis. Combined endodontic therapy and periodontal therapy or extraction are needed for the combined lesion originating with periodontal pathosis (Figs. 3–13, 3–14). Endodontic therapy alone will usually eliminate the short-lived combined lesion that originates with pulpal pathosis.

Factitial Oral Injuries

The most common causes of emergency self-inflicted traumas are floss, toothpicks, overbrushing, fingernail scratching, and water irrigators. You should anticipate that when patients start flossing some will be overzealous and floss too deeply. When you see vertical cuts into the gingiva at the line angles of teeth, suspect floss cutting (Fig. 3–15). If you suspect a patient is traumatizing the gingiva with a toothpick, let him show you how he uses it (Figs. 3–16, 3–17, 3–18). Overbrushers traumatize the gingiva and abrade the teeth at the most convex surfaces (Fig. 3–19). Initially, to eliminate discomfort, put patient on a soft brush and a different and safe brushing technique. Water irrigation normally does no damage except to give the patient a false sense of security. If, however, a patient irrigates subgingivally and senses discomfort or notices bleeding and pain, then damage is being caused. Clinical studies have shown that water irrigation can initiate tissue damage.

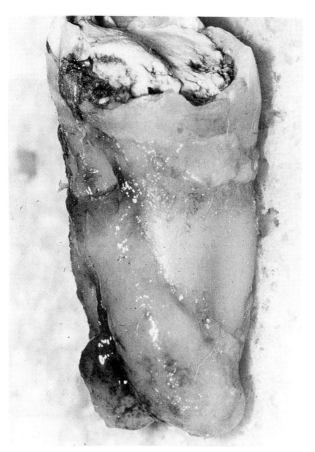

FIGURE 3–13 • An extracted tooth showing an abscess from apex moving along the root to drain through sulcus.

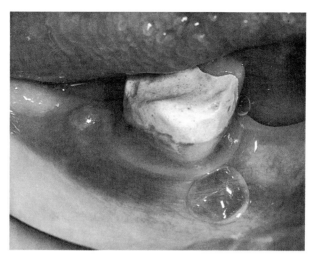

FIGURE 3–14 • Mandibular second molar with a sinus tract draining to distal. The apex could not be probed through the sulcus. Endodontic therapy eliminated the sinus tract.

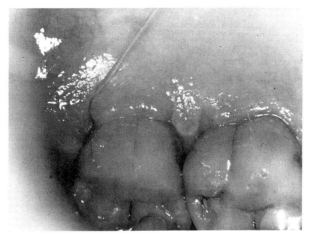

FIGURE 3–15 • Gingiva cut by improper flossing.

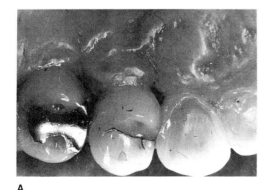
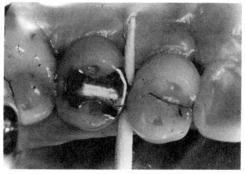

A   B

FIGURE 3–16 • Gingival trauma. (A) Trauma from unknown cause on lingual aspect. (B) Patient using a toothpick demonstrates the cause of the trauma.

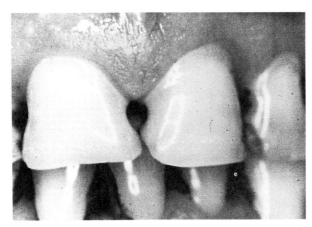

FIGURE **3–17** • Patient caused round eroded areas in maxillary anterior teeth with a toothpick used in a twirling motion.

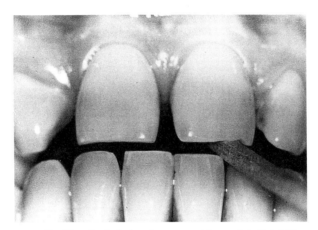

FIGURE **3–18** • Incisal abrasion caused by matchstick biting habit.

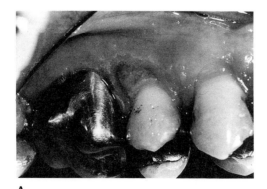
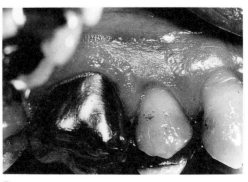

A   **B**

FIGURE **3–19** • Toothbrush trauma. (*A*) Patient presented for emergency treatment of painful ulcer on the facial aspect of the second premolar caused by toothbrush trauma. (*B*) Appearance after 10 days of using only moist cotton to clean the area.

Bibliography

Austin G, et al. The Keyes technique and self-inflicted injuries: Three case reports. J Periodontol 1985; 56:537–539.

Hallmon WW, Waldrop TC, Houston GD, Hawkins BF. Flossing clefts. Clinical and histological observations. J Periodontol 1986; 58:501–504.

Johnson BD, Engel D. Acute necrotizing ulcerative gingivitis: A review of diagnosis, etiology and treatment. J Periodontol 1986; 57:141–150.

Loesche WJ, et al. The bacteriology of acute necrotizing ulcerative gingivitis. J Periodontol 1982; 53:223–230.

Niemi ML, et al. Frequency of gingival lesions after standardized brushing as related to stiffness of toothbrush and abrasiveness of dentifrice. J Clin Periodontol 1984; 11:254–261.

Rees TD. Phenothiazine: Another possible etiologic agent in erythema multiforme: Report of a case. J Periodontol 1985; 56:480–483.

Rees TD, Orth CF. Oral ulcerations with use of hydrogen peroxide. J Periodontol 1986; 57:689–692.

Schluger S, Yuodelis RA, Page RC. Periodontal disease: Basic phenomena, clinical management, and occlusal and restorative interrelationships. Philadelphia: Lea & Febiger, 1977.

Smukler H, Landsberg J. The toothbrush and gingival traumatic injury. J Periodontol 1984; 55:713–719.

Weathers DR, Griffin JW. Intraoral ulcerations of recurrent herpes simplex and recurrent aphthae: Two distinct clinical entities. J Am Dent Assoc 1970; 81(1):81.

CHAPTER FOUR

Treatment of Gingivitis

Gingivitis (Case Type I, Code 04500) is inflammation of the gingiva. Its etiology is multifactorial, and the cause should be determined before treatment is undertaken. Although plaque-induced gingivitis is the most common type, allergies, systemic causes, hormonal influences, viruses, and self- or iatrogenically induced etiologies should be considered. In Case Type I gingivitis there is no bone loss. If bone loss is present, then a diagnosis of Case Type II or III disease should be considered. These case types are discussed in later chapters. The treatments outlined in this chapter apply only to bacterial gingivitis with no bone loss.

Most incipient or beginning gingivitis responds to effective oral hygiene and scaling (Fig. 4–1). Advanced gingivitis requires root planing as well as oral hygiene instructions. Gingival curettage may also be needed in advanced cases. It is extremely important to recognize and treat gingivitis in its early stages, since effective treatment will usually prevent progression of gingivitis to periodontitis and bone loss. Since teaching and motivating the patient to perform effective oral hygiene is the primary preventive measure in controlling gingivitis, all clinical auxillary personnel should be trained as plaque control therapists.

Scaling

Scaling is instrumentation of the crown and root surfaces of the teeth to remove plaque, calculus, and stains from these surfaces.

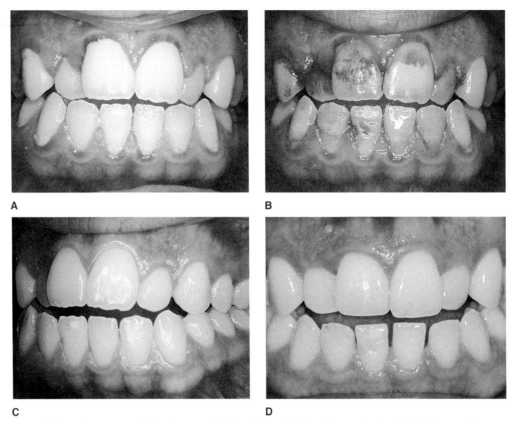

FIGURE 4–1 • Treatment of simple marginal gingivitis. (A) Simple marginal gingivitis in an 18-year-old. No calculus is present. (B) Appearance after plaque staining. The patient was given lessons in hygiene and the teeth were polished with a rubber cap. (C) Same patient after four visits. Appearance 2 months after treatment. (D) Same patient 27 years later.

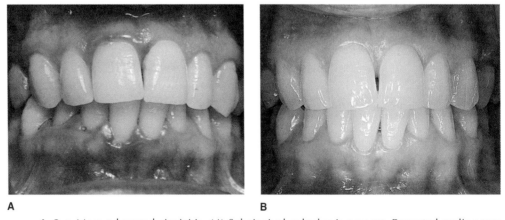

FIGURE 4–2 • More advanced gingivitis. (A) Subgingival calculus is present. Repeated scaling was performed and the patient was given instruction in oral hygiene. (B) Same patient 8 years later.

INDICATIONS FOR SCALING

1. Presence of calcified dental deposits that are not causing periodontal pathosis. Even in these circumstances, deposits should be removed as a preventive measure.
2. Presence of calcified dental deposits that are causing minimal periodontal inflammation. Even if no irreparable damage has occurred, the deposits should be removed to prevent damage (Fig. 4–2).
3. Need to eliminate gross inflammation before surgical elimination of periodontal pathosis.
4. Discovery of calcified deposits at the time of surgery.

OBJECTIVES FOR SCALING

1. To eliminate calcified and uncalcified dental deposits which are, or later may be, local irritants to the periodontal tissues.
2. To prepare the teeth for flossing.

TECHNIQUES FOR SCALING

The following instruments are used:

Ultrasonics. These are effective on visible deposits, but not as effective subgingivally.

Positive-rake instruments, such as most sickles, Jaquettes, heavy-duty scalers, and some curettes. These are effective in removing easily reached deposits attached to the tooth by bacterial plaque. They are ineffective in complete removal of deposits that extend into defects of the teeth.

Negative-rake instruments. These instruments are better than positive-rake instruments for subgingival deposits because they are thinner.

The transillumination light.

Rotary instruments. These are used only in furcations and developmental grooves where hand instrumentation is ineffective.

1. Use local anesthetics during all root instrumentation techniques when needed to prevent patient sensitivity or discomfort.
2. After instrumentation, check with the transillumination light to see if all deposits are removed. Dry the roots with air for better visualization.

Root Planing

Root planing is a definitive treatment procedure designed to remove cementum or surface dentin that is rough, impregnated with calculus, or contaminated with toxins or microorganisms (Figs. 4–3, 4–4, 4–5).

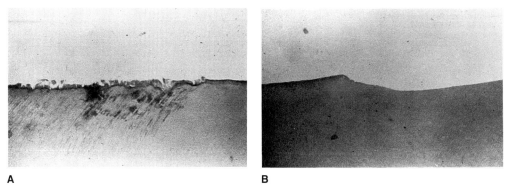

A　　　　　**B**

FIGURE **4–3** • Root planing. (A) Photomicrograph of a tooth root showing bacterial penetration into the dentinal tubules. (B) Appearance after root planing. (Courtesy Dr. T. J. O'Leary)

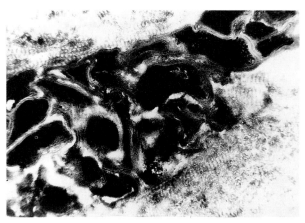

FIGURE **4–4** • Gram-positive microorganisms invading dentinal tubules in carious root dentin adjacent to a periodontal pocket. (Courtesy Dr. M. A. Listgarten)

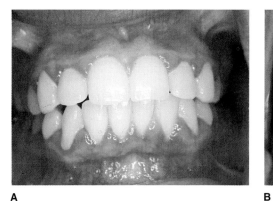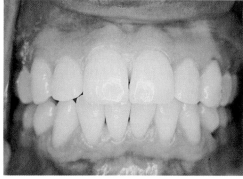

A　　　　　**B**

FIGURE **4–5** • Beginning periodontitis with no bone loss. (A) Preoperative appearance. Note the red gingival margins, bulbous papillae, and overall edematous appearance of the tissue. Treatment consisted of scaling, root planing, and curettage under local anesthesia, one quadrant at a time, home care instruction, and periodic maintenance. (B) Appearance 9 years later. Note healthy pink gingiva with knife-edge margins and firm papillae.

INDICATIONS FOR ROOT PLANING

1. Presence of deposits that have penetrated into defects of the teeth and are not removed by scaling.
2. Presence of long-standing pockets that have caused a softening of the root.
3. Presence of root roughness that harbors bacterial plaque (Fig. 4–6).

OBJECTIVES OF ROOT PLANING

1. To secure biologically acceptable root surfaces.
2. To resolve inflammation (Fig. 4–7).

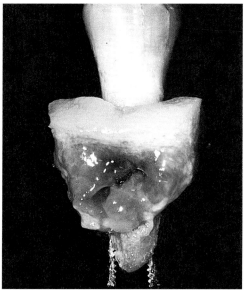 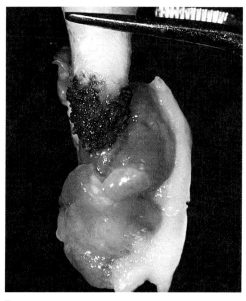

A   **B**

FIGURE **4–6** • Indications for root planing. (A) Extracted tooth with advanced periodontal pocketing. The outer surface of the gingiva looks healthy because the disease process is inside and cannot be seen. (B) Same tooth with the gingiva reflected back. Granulomatous tissue and calcified deposits are evident on the root. (Courtesy Dr. Bobby Romans)

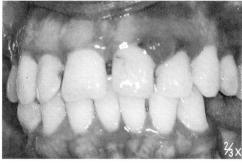 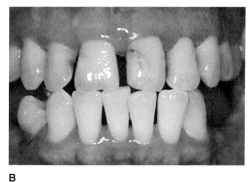

A   **B**

FIGURE **4–7** • Indications for root planing. (A) Severe gingivitis. Pockets were not sensitive on probing, so case was treated by the hygienist. Four 1-hour appointments for scaling and root planing by quadrants and plaque control instructions were used. This was followed by four half-hour plaque-control and polishing appointments. (B) Appearance 3 months later.

3. To reduce probing depths.
4. To facilitate oral hygiene procedures.
5. To improve or maintain attachment levels (Figs. 4–8, 4–9).
6. To prepare tissues for surgical procedures.

Factors influencing the effectiveness of root planing are root anatomy, pocket depth, tooth position, adequacy of the instrumentation for diagnosis or treatment, area of the mouth being treated, mouth size, elasticity of cheeks, opening range, and the dexterity of the operator.

TECHNIQUES FOR ROOT PLANING

The following instruments are used:

Files
Negative rake hoes, used after scaling (Fig. 4–10).

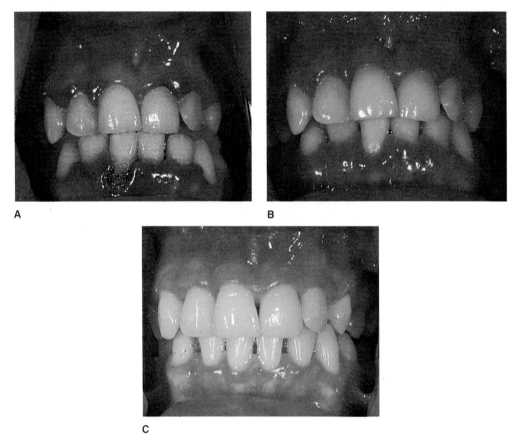

A

B

C

FIGURE 4–8 • Indications for root planing. (A) Patient with marginal gingivitis and recession on mandibular right central incisor. A regimen of scaling, root planing, and oral hygiene training was instituted. (B) Appearance 3 weeks later. (C) Appearance 3 months later. Note how gingiva has regenerated over the mandibular right central incisor. (Courtesy Dr. John M. Nabers)

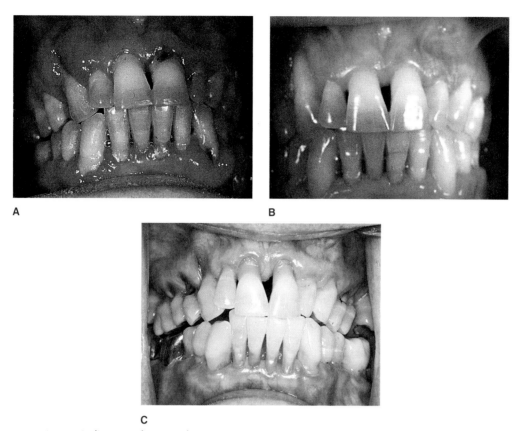

FIGURE 4–9 • Indications for root planing. (*A*) Gingivitis. The area around the maxillary right canine was excised for biopsy purposes. A regimen of multiple scalings, polishings, and oral hygiene instruction was instituted. (*B*) Appearance after treatment. (*C*) Appearance 29 years later. (Courtesy Dr. John M. Nabers)

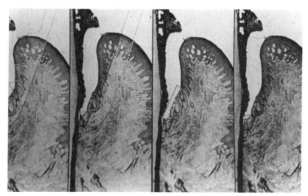

FIGURE 4–10 • Outlines of file, hoe, curette and thin sickle scaler in the periodontal pocket.

Pull-designed curettes (Fig. 4–11).
Push-designed curettes (Fig. 4–12).

1. Dry roots of teeth with air to see if the root is smooth and clean.
2. Stop to sharpen your instruments every 10 to 15 minutes: dull instruments do not clean or smooth but only burnish. They also cause operator and patient fatigue.
3. Use wrist movements in planing the roots for maximum efficiency and minimum fatigue. Finger movements cause cramping and rapid fatigue.
4. Use thumb and finger rests to maximize efficiency (Fig. 4–13).
5. Periodically monitor the smoothness of the root using a curette attached to the end of a stethoscope from which the bell has been removed. Let the patient hear the difference between a planed and an unplaned root.

Curettage

Curettage is the process of surgically debriding the soft tissue wall of a periodontal pocket.

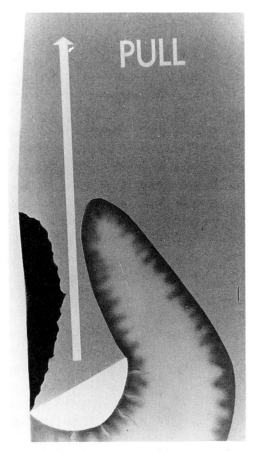

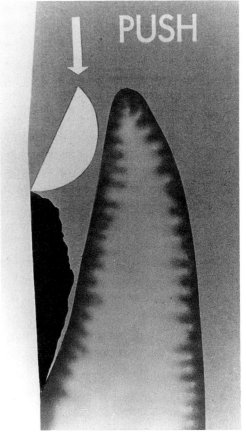

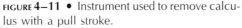

FIGURE 4–11 • Instrument used to remove calculus with a pull stroke.

FIGURE 4–12 • Instrument used to remove calculus with a push stroke.

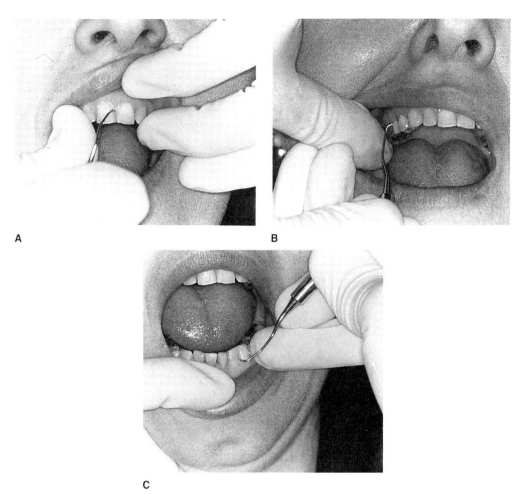

FIGURE 4–13 • Bracing techniques. (A) Thumb fulcrum rest. This position is used for maximum force on the anterior teeth. (B) Bracing finger technique. This position allows maximum stability in areas of difficult access. (C) Finger fulcrum rest. This position can be used in most areas.

INDICATIONS FOR CURETTAGE

1. Slight-to-moderate pocket depth (3–5 mm) in conjunction with soft, edematous, and fairly well contoured gingiva.
2. Appearance of an isolated new pocket in a previously treated patient. (The patient may later require resective surgery if scaling, root planing, and subgingival curettage are not effective.)

OBJECTIVES OF CURETTAGE

1. To eliminate as much of the granulomatous tissue as possible from the crevicular side of the pocket.
2. To eliminate inflammatory tissue.
3. To reduce the gingival height of the pocket by 1.0 to 2.5 mm (internal gingivectomy).
4. To remove broken interproximal papillae. Removal is followed by a papillary suture to coapt the buccal and lingual hemipapillae.

TECHNIQUE FOR CURETTAGE

1. Ensure that roots have been thoroughly planed. If they have not, curettage will be ineffective because contamination from the root surface will cause the inflammation to recur.
2. Use curettes to remove pocket lining.
3. Use coarse diamond stones on the internal side of a hemipapilla.
4. Ensure gingival coaption to teeth by applying pressure and gauze for 3 minutes. Suture if the hemipapillae are detached.

CONTROL OF HEMORRHAGE FOLLOWING CURETTAGE

Usually minor postoperative bleeding can be controlled by the patient with the use of gauze pads and pressure. If bleeding continues and a liver clot forms, anesthetize the area and remove the liver clot. If bleeding continues to be a problem, consider using electrocautery. An intramuscular injection of Synkavite (vitamin K) has proved beneficial in cases where postoperative bleeding is a particular problem.

Followup Treatment

After scaling, root planing, or curettage is completed, wait about 6 weeks to allow time for tissue healing, resolution of edema, and restoration of normal gingival contours before proceeding with more advanced treatments. If tissues are highly inflamed and edematous, scaling and root planing may be all that is required to achieve resolution. If there is fibrous pocket tissue, resolution would not be expected.

Plan on a re-evaluation of the patient's periodontal status during initial treatment planning. This will prevent misunderstandings between you and the patient as treatment progresses. Providing the patient with a copy of the treatment plan will help in this regard. Some doctors have patients initial the treatment plan to indicate understanding. The treatment plan should be written in lay terms.

Bibliography

Adriaens PA, et al. Ultrastructural observations on bacterial invasion in cementum and radicular dentin of periodontally diseased human teeth. J Periodontol 1988; 59:493–503.

Aleo JJ, et al. The presence and biologic activity of cementum-bound endotoxin. J Periodontol 1974; 45:672–675.

Baderstein A, et al. Effect of nonsurgical periodontal therapy. III. Single versus repeated instrumentation. J Clin Periodontol 1984; 11:114–124.

Benfenati MP, et al. Scanning electron microscope: An SEM study of periodontally instrumented root surfaces, comparing sharp, dull, and damaged curettes and ultrasonic instruments. Int J Periodont Res Dent 1987; 2:51–68.

Daly CG, et al. Histological assessment of periodontally involved cementum. J Clin Periodontol 9:266–274, 1982.

Garrett JS. Root planing: A perspective. J Periodontol 1977; 48:553–557.

Hatfield CG, Baumhammers A. Cytotoxic effects of periodontally involved surfaces of human teeth. Arch Oral Biol 1971; 16:465–468.

Isidor F, et al. The effect of root planing as compared to that of surgical treatment. J Clin Periodontol 1984; 11:669–681.

Lindhe J, et al. Scaling and root planing in shallow pockets. J Clin Periodontol 1982; 9:415–418.

Magnusson I, et al. Recolonization of a subgingival microbiota following scaling in deep pockets. J Clin Periodontol 1984; 11:193–207.

O'Leary TJ. The impact of research on scaling and root planing. J Periodontol 1986; 57:69–75.

Selvig KA. Attachment of plaque and calculus to tooth surfaces. J Periodontol Res 1970; 5:8–18.

Stahl SS, et al. Soft tissue healing following curettage and root planing. J Periodontol 1971; 42:678–684.

Waerhaug J. Healing of the dento-epithelial junction following subgingival plaque control. J Periodontol 1978; 49:1–10.

Wilkinson RF, Maybury JE. Scanning electron microscopy of the root surface following instrumentation. J Periodontol 1973; 44:559–563.

CHAPTER FIVE

Treatment of Early Periodontitis

Early periodontitis (moderate pockets with minor bone loss [Case Type II Code 04600]) sometimes responds to the treatment already described for gingivitis. If the tissues are soft and edematous, the chances are good that with thorough conservative treatment the pockets will be eliminated without resective surgery. If, however, the pockets persist, then surgical resection must be considered.

Gingivectomy and Gingivoplasty

Gingivectomy is defined as the excision of the soft-tissue wall of the periodontal pocket. Gingivoplasty is a surgical procedure used to reshape the tissue in order to create a normal, functional form.

These procedures were used extensively in the past in periodontics. They are relatively fast and simple techniques which are ideal for the situations in which they are indicated.

INDICATIONS FOR GINGIVECTOMY AND GINGIVOPLASTY

1. Normal bone height and contours, but fibrous hyperplasia of the gingiva.
2. Acceptable bone contours, but slight bone loss with fibrous gingival pockets of 3 to 5 mm. Sufficient attached gingiva must be present to allow physiological contouring during surgery. All incisions will be in attached gingiva.
3. Chronic soft-tissue craters or clefts with abundant attached gingivae.

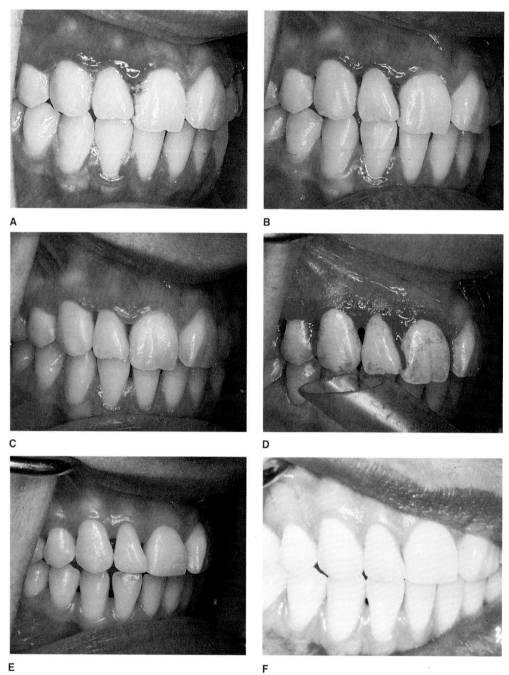

FIGURE **5–1** • Treatment of acute necrotizing ulcerative gingivitis. (*A*) Appearance on first appointment. Scaling and debridement was performed. (*B*) Appearance one day later. (*C*) Appearance after initial healing. Note bulbous contours and flaps of detached tissue. (*D*) Gingivoplasty performed 6 weeks after initial therapy. Note the deflecting contours, scalloped architectural form, pointed papillae, and parallel cemento-enamel junction. (*E*) Same case, 6 weeks later. Note the interproximal embrasure spaces. (*F*) Appearance 27 years later.

OBJECTIVES OF GINGIVECTOMY AND GINGIVOPLASTY

1. To eliminate fibrous hyperplasia of the gingiva, to restore normal contours (Fig. 5–1), and to minimize crevicular depth.
2. To eliminate pockets by removing diseased tissues, to create normal contours, and to establish a result that is cleanable to prevent further bone loss.
3. To eliminate soft-tissue craters and defects.

Gingivectomy and/or gingivoplasty is contraindicated when the base of pocket is apical to the mucogingival junction, because in this case there would not be an adequate zone of functional gingiva after surgery.

TECHNIQUE FOR GINGIVECTOMY

1. Use a scalloped incision around the roots, keeping it as parallel as possible to cemento-enamel junctions (Fig. 5–2).
2. Remove any tissue tags.

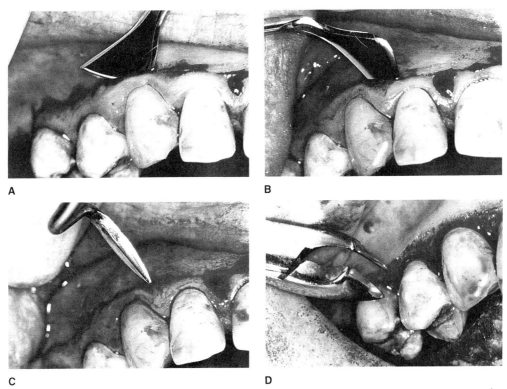

FIGURE 5–2 • Gingivectomy. (A) Initial incision, using a Kirkland 15k/16k knife. (B) Starting the interproximal incision, using a Kirkland 15k/16k knife. (C) Finishing the interproximal incisions. Orban 1 and 2 knives are used because of their thinness. (D) Surgical nippers are used to accentuate the interdental grooving and to remove tissue tags.

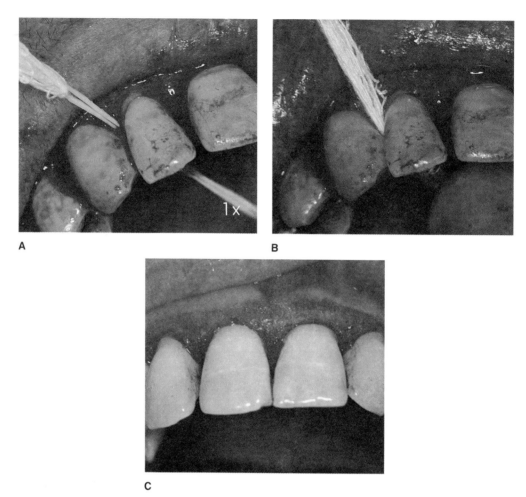

A

B

C

FIGURE 5–3 • Gingivectomy. Contouring the papillae. (A) Floss threader with gauze attached is inserted interproximally. (B) The gauze is sawed back and forth to polish the incised area. This helps eliminate tissue tags. (C) Appearance after use of gauze. Note the scalloped line on each tooth with deflecting contours and pointed papillae. There are no osseous exposures.

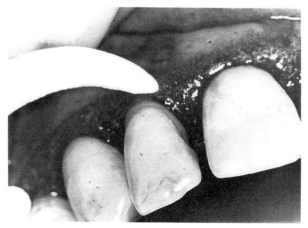

FIGURE 5–4 • Gingivectomy. Scaling is best done during surgery while teeth are anesthetized.

3. Contour the papillae so that food will be deflected away from the teeth.
4. Use gauze to smooth the surgical wound (Fig. 5–3).
5. Perform thorough scaling and root planing at the time of surgery while the teeth are anesthetized (Fig. 5–4).
6. Polish the incised surface with gauze.
7. Place protective dressings (Fig. 5–5).
8. Change dressings every 4 to 7 days until the incision is healed to the point of complete epithelial coverage.
9. Chemically cauterize any areas of granulation overgrowth (Fig. 5–6).
10. Have the patient use chlorhexidine mouth rinses twice daily for 2 weeks after the last dressing removal.
11. Polish the teeth and review home care procedures when the last dressing is removed.
12. Scale and root plane if any deposit is visible or a localized area has not healed properly.

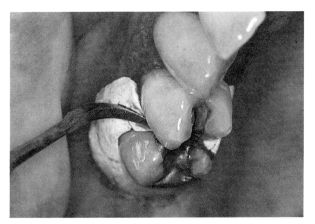

FIGURE 5–5 • Gingivectomy. Placement of surgical dressing interproximally.

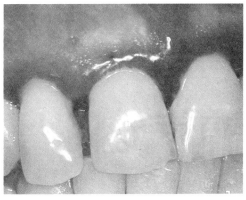
A

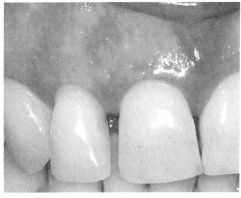
B

FIGURE 5–6 • Gingivectomy. (A) Appearance 2 weeks after surgery. (B) Appearance at completion of treatment 2 months later.

13. As with any surgical procedure, use local anesthetics as required to prevent patient discomfort. Nerve blocks are more effective than infiltration anesthesia.
14. Repolish the teeth every 2 or 3 weeks and check plaque control until the desired result is obtained (6 to 12 weeks after final dressing removal).

The various surgical procedures discussed in the rest of this chapter and the beginning of the next chapter are very similar, and their differences need to be delineated to avoid confusion. These procedures are generally used to treat Case Type III (Code 04700) as well as Case Type II (Code 04600) cases.

Excisional New Attachment Procedure

The excisional new attachment procedure (ENAP) is a surgical procedure in which an internal bevel incision is made to remove the crevicular lining and junctional epithelium in the treatment of mild-to-moderate periodontal pockets. The goal of the procedure is removal of the epithelial lining of the pocket to allow the possibility of new attachment. The procedure also allows access for root preparation.

In the past this procedure was known as the Mini Flap. ENAP is not a flap procedure, however, but a subgingival curettage with a knife. The incision is made from the crest of the free gingiva to the base of the epithelial attachment to the root. No flap is reflected.

INDICATIONS FOR ENAP

1. Slight bone loss with slight-to-moderate pocketing (3 to 5 mm) and a need to avoid exposure of excision. The procedure is used primarily in the maxillary anterior region, particularly in patients who have a high lip-line smile showing a lot of gingiva.
2. Suprabony pockets whose base is not apical to the mucogingival junction.

OBJECTIVES OF ENAP

1. To avoid long-looking teeth resulting from excisional gingival resections.
2. To assure removal of the pocket lining and obtain better access for root preparation.
3. To obtain new attachment.

TECHNIQUE FOR ENAP

1. Use a Bard-Parker #11 or #12 blade for incisions.
2. Remove the internal collar of tissues and tissue tabs.
3. Scale and root plane the roots adjacent to the pocket.
4. Coapt tissues back to the teeth with interrupted interproximal sutures.
5. Hold flaps in place with saline-soaked gauze using light pressure for 3 minutes.

6. Place protective dressing.
7. Remove dressing and sutures in 7 days.
8. Use a cotton applicator stick soaked with 1–2% hydrogen peroxide to clean the area.
9. If the patient is sensitive to cleaning, or if the wound bleeds, replace dressing for one more week.
10. Have the patient use chlorhexidine mouth rinse twice daily for 2 weeks after last dressing removal.
11. When the dressing is removed, polish the teeth and review home care procedures. The patient may have to use large cotton balls soaked with warm water to clean the operated area for a few days before brushing.
12. Scale and root plane any isolated roots where healing is delayed.
13. Cauterize any areas of granulation overgrowth with trichloroacetic acid and neutralize with isopropyl alcohol. This cautery is self-limiting and will not cause deeper destruction.

Full-Thickness and Partial-Thickness Flaps

The only difference between a partial-thickness flap and a full-thickness flap is the preoperative thickness of the gingiva to be flapped. If the gingiva is excessively thick, the incision should be made parallel to the tooth so that the gingival flap is no more than 1.5 mm thick. If the bone covering the roots appears to be thin, the mucoperiosteum should not be reflected because exposing bone is likely to result in a bony dehiscence.

Modified Widman Flap

The modified Widman procedure is a replaced mucoperiosteal flap procedure which has reattachment of the gingiva to the tooth as its goal. It is designed to retain a maximum amount of gingival tissue while allowing access to roots and bone.

INDICATIONS FOR THE MODIFIED WIDMAN FLAP

1. Deep pockets.
2. Intrabony pockets.
3. Need to minimize recession, as in the anterior regions (Fig. 5–7A).

ADVANTAGES OF THE MODIFIED WIDMAN FLAP

1. There is intimate postoperative coaptation of healthy collagenous tissues to all tooth surfaces. (A long junctional epithelial attachment may develop.)
2. Bone is conserved.
3. There is soft-tissue coverage of root surfaces, which conserves esthetics, facilitates oral hygiene, and decreases the root's sensitivity and susceptibility to caries.
4. Postoperative pain and discomfort are minimal.

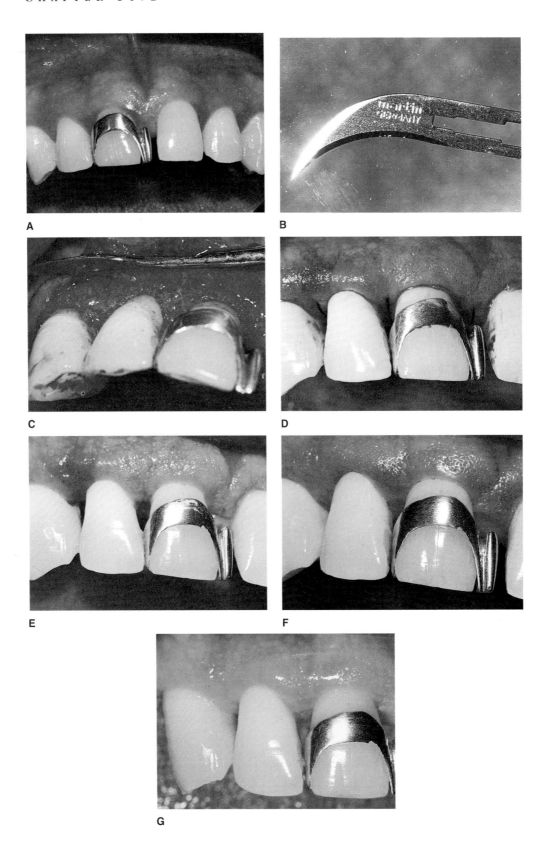

A

B

C

D

E

F

G

FIGURE 5–7 • Modified Widman flap procedure. (A) Preoperative view of patient with inflamed pockets in maxillary anterior tooth. (B) Martin #12b blade used to incise tissues. (C) Access to roots and bone for thorough debridement. (D) Primary closure with minimum tissue reduction. (E) Appearance 1 week after surgery. Note necrosis of interdental closure areas. (F) Appearance 3 months after surgery. The interdental areas are regenerating. (G) Appearance 12 months after surgery. The interdental areas have healed. The labial tissues have receded because of resolution of inflammation.

DISADVANTAGES OF THE MODIFIED WIDMAN FLAP

1. Reattachment may not occur, resulting in pocket recurrence.
2. The technique is demanding and will fail if primary closure with good tissue-tooth coaptation is not achieved.
3. There will still be some postoperative tissue shrinkage once healing occurs.

TECHNIQUE FOR THE MODIFIED WIDMAN FLAP

1. Use a #11 or #12b blade for incisions (Fig. 5–7B).
2. Direct the first incision parallel to the long axis of the tooth, 0.5–1 mm buccal and lingual from the free gingival margin (Fig. 5–8). Use an

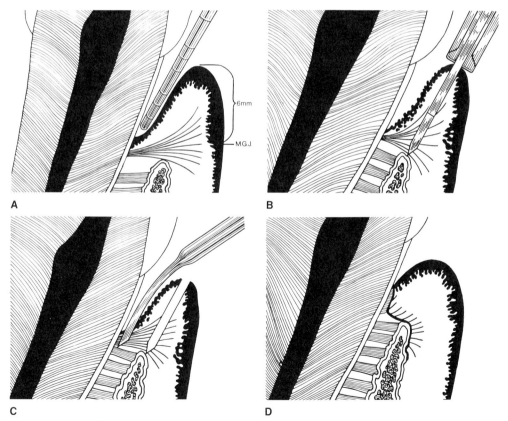

FIGURE 5–8 • Widman flap procedure. (A) Diagram of 6-mm pocket. *MGJ*, mucogingival junction. (B) Incision parallel to long axis of tooth directed to the alveolar crest. (C) Incision to free internal collar of tissue. (D) Flap closure. (Courtesy Dr. Peter Fedi)

intracrevicular incision if pockets are shallow or esthetics are critical. This may require a reverse bevel and exaggerated scalloping on the palatal or lingual aspect to achieve primary closure. Primary closure is essential to success, so as little interproximal tissue as possible should be removed.

3. Make vertical releasing incisions through the interdental papillae 2–3 mm apical to the initial incisions.
4. Make the next incision around the neck of each tooth parallel to the long axis to the alveolar bone.
5. Make a last incision to cut loose the collar of tissue left around the tooth (Fig. 5–8C).
6. Carefully plane root surfaces to remove all plaque and calculus. Do not remove any healthy periodontal ligament fibers (see Fig. 5–7C).
7. Remove soft tissues from the exposed alveolar bone.
8. Irrigate the area with sterile saline.
9. Coapt the flaps to ensure primary closure interproximally and close coaptation to the teeth. Flap thinning or bone recontouring may be necessary to accomplish this (see Fig. 5–7D).
10. Close the flaps, using interrupted 4-0 black silk sutures and an FS-2 needle. Incomplete closure of flaps often gives poor results, such as residual pockets and inflamed tissues.
11. Dress the area with a periodontal dressing for 1 week. Remove the dressing and sutures if healing is complete in 7 days. If not, redress and wait another 5–7 days for dressing removal. Have the patient rinse with 0.12% chlorhexidine mouth rinse twice daily for 2 weeks after the last dressing removal.
12. Polish teeth and review home care instructions after suture removal. There may be shallow interproximal craters initially; plaque control is critical until these areas fill in (Fig. 5–7 E–G). The chlorhexidine will help considerably in this regard.

Apically Positioned Flap (APF)

When a pocket extends so far that its base is near or apical to the mucogingival junction, it creates difficult treatment problems. Alveolar mucosa is structurally and functionally quite different from gingiva. Any attempt to make alveolar mucosa serve the function of gingiva would result in a gaping, slow-healing wound, a considerable amount of pain for the patient, a gingival margin covered by tissue ill-suited to its purpose, and a doubtful prognosis. The APF procedure, as its name suggests, is designed to reposition a flap of gingiva apically, thereby avoiding the complications that would arise from the replacement of gingiva by alveolar mucosa.

Attached gingiva has a very dense collagenous, fibrous connective tissue and is firmly attached to the underlying tooth surface and to bone. There are no elastic connective tissue fibers in attached gingiva. The alveolar mucosa, on the other hand, has a loose submucosa, which is rich in elastic tissue. When incised, the elastic tissues retract, leaving a gaping wound. Also, there is a difference in the surface epithelium covering these two different tissues. The attached gingiva is covered by a heavy stratified squamous epithelium with long epithelial ridges and is well keratinized on the surface. The epithelium of the alveolar mucosa is rather thin, has no ridges, and is nonkeratinized. Masticatory mucosa, then, is especially adapted to withstand the trauma of masticatory stresses. The attached gingiva is designed for the function of mastication, whereas the alveolar mucosa is designed for the function of lining the oral cavity, keeping it moist and smooth. Its surface cannot withstand the friction of food during mastication. If alveolar mucosa is made to serve in the place of gingiva, the newly established gingival margin will be covered by a tissue not adapted to its functional requirements and injury in mastication will occur. Oral hygiene procedures for this area will be difficult if not impossible, since brushing can be painful. The prognosis for such a procedure would be at least very doubtful. The APF procedure was developed to avoid these difficulties. Use of the procedure in properly selected cases allows for the elimination of pockets and long-term retention of the teeth.

INDICATIONS FOR APF

1. A pocket that extends to or apical to the mucogingival junction.
2. A moderate chronic pocket that is to be eliminated in conjunction with osseous surgery in which the postoperative bone margin will be apical to the preoperative mucogingival junction.

OBJECTIVES OF APF

1. In a pocket that extends to the mucogingival junction: to eliminate the diseased tissues; to eliminate the pocket; and to save the mature functional gingival tissue to graft into a new position apical to where the gingiva was originally. This is necessary in order that the gingiva can attach to the bone and roots of the teeth.
2. To obtain access for osseous contouring intended to eliminate minor bony defects not amenable to bone-fill repair.
3. To achieve a healed normal interrelationship between gingivae, teeth, and bone.
4. To create a covering for contoured bone. This bone is a living, sensitive tissue and a prepared gingival graft is more physiologically acceptable than anything else.

TECHNIQUE FOR APF

1. If the gingiva to be repositioned is thin, make the initial incision through the labial, lingual, or buccal crevices to the bone (crevicular incision). Tailor this incision in a scalloped contour so that complete coverage of bone is possible. If only a small area is involved, a lateral vertical incision into the mucosa at one or both ends gives better access. Remove the crevicular epithelium physically with a rotary instrument or hand instrumentation.
2. If the gingiva is thick or abundant, use a partial-thickness incision within the gingiva to ease deflection, thin the gingiva, and excise the crevicular epithelium, epithelial attachment, and inflammatory tissues (Fig. 5–9).

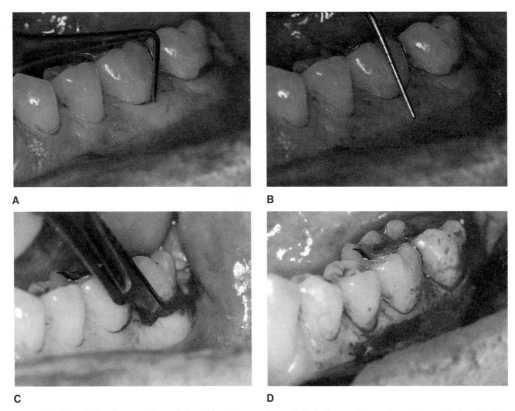

FIGURE 5–9 • Apically positioned flap (APF) procedure. (*A*) A 6-mm buccal pocket with beginning furcation involvement is apparent. (*B*) Patient has 3 mm of masticatory mucosa (gingiva). The tip of the probe is at the mucogingival junction. (*C*) A vertical incision is made with a Bard-Parker #15 blade, creating a very thin retained gingival flap. (*D*) The remaining tissues next to the tooth will be excised to eliminate the pockets.

3. After completing any indicated osseous contouring, suture the gingiva back loosely so that the incisal edge of the gingiva can be positioned at or near the bone margin. Thus, the retained gingiva is now positioned on bone. Use periosteal suturing to place the gingiva precisely in the desired position (Fig. 5–10).

4. Always probe at the interface between the retained gingiva and the root until you touch the crest of the bone. This interface should not be over 1 to 1.5 mm if complete pocket elimination is desired. If the interface depth is greater than 1.5 mm, resuture and/or recontour the gingival flap to correct this situation.

5. After placing interrupted interproximal sutures, hold the flap in position with gauze for 2 or 3 minutes to stop bleeding and to obtain a thin fibrin clot. This helps to hold the flap in its position.

6. Place compressed Gelfoam, shaped to cover the interproximal suture and any exposed bone, and cover with a dressing. The Gelfoam keeps the dressing away from the suture knots and any exposed bone. The objective is to leave a clot between the bone and the dressing. This clot will later be replaced by granulation tissue and in time will become functional gingiva (see Fig. 5–10 B–D).

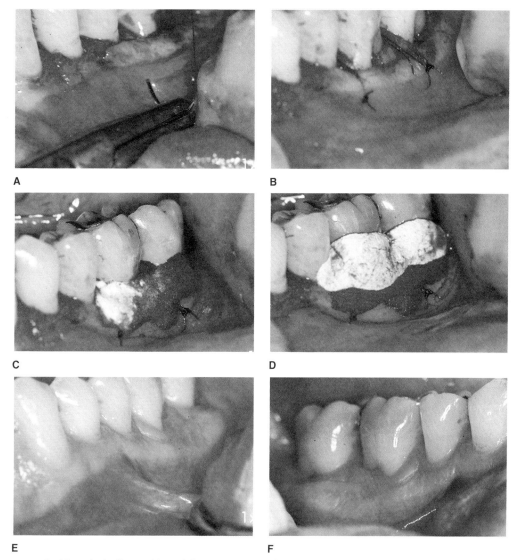

FIGURE **5−10** • Apically positioned flap (APF) procedure. Suturing technique. (A) An atraumatic suture is placed through the alveolar mucosa and periosteum. (B) Double interproximal sutures are placed. The periosteal suture holds the tissue in proper apical position. The gingival suture holds the tissue against the bone. Note the exposed bone. (C) Gelfoam mixed with the patient's blood is placed over exposed bone to prevent dressings from touching the living sensitive bone tissue. (D) Dressing covering Gelfoam. (E) At final healing note old/new gingival junction and amount of new attached gingiva present. (F) Mirror view of same area, showing healthy pointed papillae tucked into the furcas.

7. Change dressings every 5 to 7 days until healing has progressed to the point of complete epithelialization (usually 10 to 14 days after surgery, depending on the area of healing and the patient's healing capacity). Remove sutures between 5 and 10 days after surgery.
8. Have the patient rinse twice daily with a 0.12% chlorhexidine mouth rinse for 2 weeks after removal of the dressing.

Postoperative Instructions

Postoperative instructions for patients are shown in Table 5–1. You should discuss these instructions in detail with the patient before dismissal and give the patient a copy to refer to. Our policy has been to call each patient in the evening after surgery. This gives the patient a chance to let you know if there are any problems. It has also proven to be a good practice-building technique.

Table 5–1 • POSTOPERATIVE INSTRUCTIONS FOR PERIODONTAL PATIENTS

General Instructions

1. Do not rinse vigorously in the first 2 hours and avoid exertion in the first 24 hours.
2. While lips and tongue are numb, be careful not to bite them or push on any protective dressing.
3. The day after surgery, use warm salt water (½ tsp. salt dissolved in 8 oz. warm water) to lightly rinse after each meal and before bedtime.
4. The day after surgery, floss and brush areas not operated.
5. On the fourth day after surgery, floss and brush operated areas not covered with a dressing.
6. Do not use water spray devices.

Diet

Adequate nutrition is essential for normal healing. Fresh vegetables or fruits can be liquefied in a blender to avoid the pressures of chewing. Nutrament, Sego, Carnation Instant Breakfast, etc., are also excellent liquid diets. Do *not* miss any meals or you will have more pain. Do not chew solid foods on areas where there are dressings. You can have *tepid* liquids such as soup, malts, Nutrament, etc., when the numbness leaves your lips. Take nothing ice-cold for at least 2 hours after surgery. *Do eat well* before you come in for a dressing change appointment as you will not be able to eat for 3 hours after a dressing change.

Pain

An ice bag may be applied to the face for 20 minutes on and 20 minutes off to help control pain and swelling. (Repeat the same procedure again in 1 hour.) Some swelling is to be expected. Avoid clenching or gritting the teeth, as pressures on the teeth will cause pain. Report any uncontrollable pain so that corrective measures can be taken.

Medications

1. Do *not* drive an automobile or work near dangerous machinery, sewing machines, power saws, etc., for at least 8 hours after taking prescribed medications for pain.
2. Do *not* drink alcoholic beverages while taking any medications.
3. Do *not* take aspirin or aspirin-containing medications for 1 week after surgery as they cause postoperative bleeding for some people.

Table 5–1 • POSTOPERATIVE INSTRUCTIONS FOR PERIODONTAL PATIENTS (CONTINUED)

Medications

4. Use prescribed pain medication, if needed.
5. Take pain medications with food to prevent possible nausea.
6. If antibiotics are prescribed, take them as directed until all have been taken. Do not drink milk or take calcium within 2 hours of taking antibiotics, if taking tetracycline.
7. Report any nausea or allergic reaction that may develop.
8. After finishing antibiotics, drink buttermilk or eat yogurt daily for 3 days to replace good bacteria in the intestines that may have been killed by the antibiotics.

Bleeding

Slow oozing is normal for several hours. One drop of blood will discolor saliva to a light red color. If bleeding is excessive:
1. Apply dry gauze or a tea bag moistened in warm water on each side of bleeding area and hold with pressure for 30 minutes. Repeat if necessary.
2. Place an ice bag against cheek or jaw for 20 minutes.
3. Sit up in bed or prop head up with two or three pillows.
4. If bleeding continues, call the office or the home telephone number listed at the bottom of this page. [Doctor's home number would be on instruction sheet.]

Loss of Protective Dressing

Loss of any part of the protective dressing is not a problem unless it causes you pain or discomfort, in which case you should call the office. We will remove any sutures at the proper time. Do not be concerned if you see white areas around the edges of the dressing.

Bibliography

Barrington EP. An overview of periodontal surgical procedures. J Periodontol 1981; 52:518–528.

Becker N, et al. A longitudinal study comparing scaling, osseous surgery, and modified Widman procedures: Results after one year. J Periodontol 1988; 59:351–365.

Cohen, Edward. Atlas of periodontal surgery. Philadelphia: Lea & Febiger, 1988.

Glickman I, Imber LR. Comparison of gingival resection with electrosurgery and periodontal knives—a biometric and histologic study. J Periodontol 1970; 41:142–148.

Kakehashi S, Parakkal PF. Proceedings from the State of the Art Workshop on Surgical Therapy for Periodontitis. 1982; 53:475–501.

Kaldahl WB, et al. Evaluation of four modalities of periodontal therapy. J Periodontol 1988; 59:783–793.

Minutello JS, et al. Evaluation of preoperative Diflunisal for postoperative pain following periodontal surgery. J Periodontol 1988; 59:390–393.

Nabers, CL. Repositioning the attached gingiva. J Periodontol 1954; 25:38–39.

Peng TK, et al. The regeneration of gingival basement membrane antigens during second wound healing. J Periodontol 1985; 56:426–429.

Ramfjord SP, Nissle RR. The modified Widman flap. J Periodontol 1974; 45:601–607.

Smith BA, et al. Mucoperiosteal flaps with and without removal of the pocket epithelium. J Periodontol 1987; 58:78–85.

Yukna RA, et al. Clinical study of healing in humans following the excisional new attachment procedure. J Periodontol 1976; 47:696–700.

Yukna RA, Williams JE. Five year evaluation of the excisional new attachment procedure. J Periodontol 1980; 51:382–385.

Yukna RA, Lawrence JJ. Gingival surgery for soft tissue new attachment. Dent Clin North Am 1980; 24:705–718.

CHAPTER SIX

Treatment of
Moderate Periodontitis

Moderate periodontitis (Case Type III Code 04700) is characterized by moderate-to-deep pockets, moderate-to-severe bone loss, and unsatisfactory topography. The condition requires either extensive treatment procedures or a compromise holding program. The latter—consisting of periodic scaling and root planing—is indicated if the patient is not at least 80% effective in plaque control, has medical complications, is emotionally unstable, is an uncontrollable alcoholic, or cannot afford complete treatment, but does want to save his teeth. Definitive treatment consists of the procedures described here. Some of the procedures described for treatment of Case Type II may also be used for Case Type III treatments. These are the ENAP, modified Widman flap, and apically positioned flap procedures.

Flap Curettage

Flap curettage is very similar to the modified Widman flap. It is intended, however, to be used when pockets are deeper and there is more bone loss. It is the initial flap design normally used when regenerative procedures are being attempted.

INDICATIONS FOR FLAP CURETTAGE

1. Acute periodontal abscess that has caused rapid bone loss.
2. Chronic deep vertical pockets with three-wall bony morphology.
3. Chronic moderate pockets with osseous defects of over 5 mm depth where osseous grafting will probably be performed.

4. Maxillary anteriors where long teeth would show postoperatively and be a source of cosmetic embarrassment.

OBJECTIVES OF FLAP CURETTAGE

1. To obtain access for the first two indications listed above with complete closure to protect the area for potential bone-fill repair.
2. To obtain access for the third indication listed above so that the patient's own mature gingival tissue can provide the coverage for the grafted site.
3. To prevent the appearance of extremely long teeth postoperatively.
   NOTE: Many times the gingiva will slowly recede back after operation to the point that it will appear that a gingivectomy or apically repositioned gingival graft flap has been done. If a long junctional epithelial attachment is obtained, excellent care is essential to prevent rapidly developing new pockets. It is much easier to maintain good health in long soft-tissue attachments in the anterior segment than in the posterior areas.

TECHNIQUE FOR FLAP CURETTAGE

1. Make a crevicular incision through the labial and/or lingual crevices to the bone, retaining as much of the interdental papilla as possible. If a restricted area is being flapped, a vertical incision at one or both ends to the mucogingival junction or into the mucosa is needed to reflect the flap adequately (Fig. 6–1 A,B).
2. Remove any inflammatory tissue and epithelial lining using scissors, knives, or coarse diamond stones (Fig. 6–1 C).
3. Suture after scaling, root planing, or osseous contouring to close or coapt the wound. Sterile normal saline is the irrigant of choice because it has no contaminants (Fig. 6–1 D,E). A dressing may not be needed if the wound is completely closed.
4. Hold a saline-soaked gauze under pressure for 2 or 3 minutes to stick the flap into position and stop bleeding while developing an initial fibrous adhesion through a thin clot.
5. If osseous exposure exists, place Gelfoam under the interproximal sutures over the bone.
6. Place Gelfoam or orabase ointment over suture knots to prevent suture incorporation into surgical dressing.
7. Remove sutures on the 5th to 7th day and start patient on twice-daily 0.12% chlorhexidine rinses.
8. Start the patient on oral hygiene procedures after dressing removal (Fig. 6–1 F).

Osseous Contouring

Osseous contouring is the excision of alveolar bone to reshape deformities caused by periodontitis and restore normal bony contours to the alveolus (Fig. 6–2).

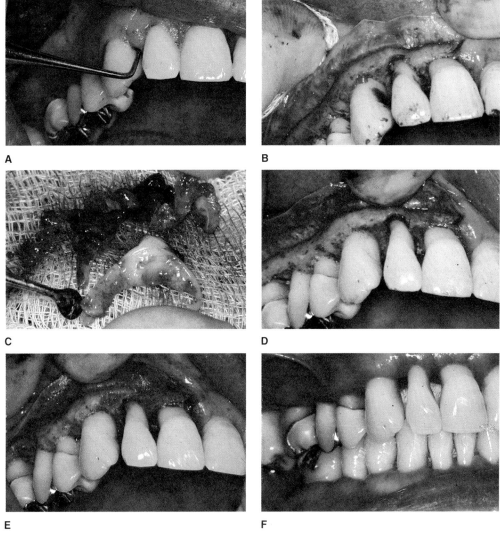

FIGURE 6–1 • Flap curettage. (A) Probe and healthy-looking gingiva. (B) Full flap reflected. Osseous defects and calcified subgingival deposits are apparent. These were smooth because of periodic scalings performed by a doctor who did not believe in surgical treatment. (C) Diseased tissues removed during the operation on this quadrant. This tissue was not visible before surgery as it was not exposed. (D) Appearance after scaling and root planing. (E) Interdental grooves cut in bone to create deflecting contours. No bone was removed that helped support the teeth. The rotary instruments used to resculpture the bone were irrigated copiously with sterile normal saline. (F) Postoperative result. With pockets eliminated, the patient can now clean all of the teeth.

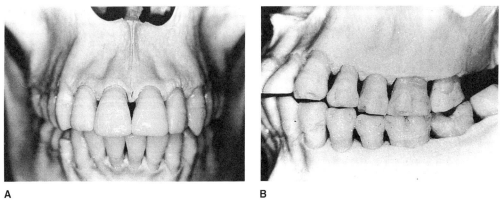

FIGURE 6–2 • Normal bone contours. (A) Around the anterior teeth. On each tooth there is a scalloped contour that parallels the cemento-enamel junction (CEJ). The interproximal bone contour is conical. (B) Around the posterior teeth. The premolar interproximal bone contour is spherical but becomes flatter posterior to the first molar. Normally the bone parallels the CEJ on the posterior teeth also.

87

INDICATIONS FOR OSSEOUS CONTOURING

1. Slight-to-moderate chronic osseous defects.
2. Beginning furcation involvements.
3. Pockets that have advanced until tori, exostosis, or shelves are involved, coronal to the base of the pocket.

OBJECTIVES OF OSSEOUS CONTOURING

1. To eliminate chronic pockets and to create tissue contours that can be maintained by the patient's oral hygiene.
2. To eliminate osseous contours associated with furcation involvements, thereby creating healed deflecting contours.
3. To eliminate tori, exostosis, shelves, and pockets and to create physiological contours that are easier for the patient to clean and maintain.
4. To create contours that can better withstand food flow pressures during mastication.

TECHNIQUE FOR OSSEOUS CONTOURING

1. Always use sterile procedures: use sterile gloves and caps and autoclaved instruments, wash the patient's face thoroughly, and have the patient rinse with chlorhexidine before starting.
2. Gain access by a flap (Fig. 6–3).
3. Use rotary instruments to remove bulky portions of bone.
4. Drip or spray sterile normal saline on any rotary instrument used on bone to avoid dehydration and overheating, which may cause bone necrosis.

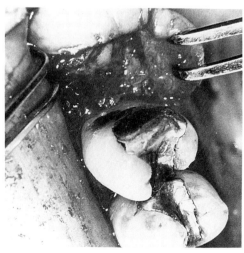 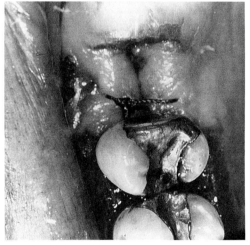

A   **B**

FIGURE 6–3 • Osseous contouring. (A) Distal osseous crater. A minimal amount of buccal and lingual osseous tissue was removed to create a physiologic architectural form in the bone to parallel the cemento-enamel junction. (B) Primary closure of the buccal and lingual flaps after the distal wedge of tissue had been removed.

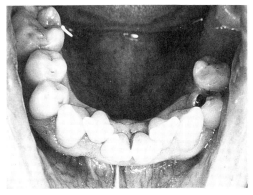
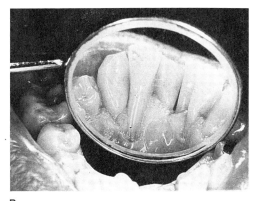

A   B

FIGURE **6–4** • Indications for lateral pedicle gingival graft. (*A*) Lateral incisors in lingual version. (*B*) Lingual view of lateral incisors of same patient shows advanced recessions of the bone and gingiva (alveolar dehiscence). This often occurs on teeth severely malposed.

5. Use hand chisels, files, or rongeurs to remove bone adjacent to a tooth so that the root will not be damaged.
6. Place any osseous material removed from the patient into a sterile dappen dish containing sterile isotonic saline. This will be used as osseous coagulum graft material if needed.
7. Close with sutures following the technique described for the flap or apically positioned flap procedures. Be careful to cover all exposed bone with gingival tissue or Gelfoam (Fig. 6–3 B).

Lateral Pedicle Gingival Graft

The lateral pedicle gingival graft is a graft elevated from a donor site, to which it remains attached at its base for nourishment, and transferred to an adjacent recipient site.

INDICATIONS FOR THE LATERAL PEDICLE GINGIVAL GRAFT

1. Deep gingival recession associated with an alveolar dehiscence or mucogingival pocket problem (Fig. 6–4).
2. Need to cover exposed root for cosmetic reasons.

REQUIREMENTS FOR THE LATERAL PEDICLE GINGIVAL GRAFT

1. Adequate adjacent tissue to develop the flap must exist.
2. The donor gingiva should be fairly thick. It should not be from a tooth with alveolar dehiscence.

OBJECTIVE OF THE LATERAL PEDICLE GINGIVAL GRAFT

1. To cover the involved root with a gingival graft in order to eliminate the defect.

TECHNIQUE FOR THE LATERAL PEDICLE GINGIVAL GRAFT

1. Prepare the recipient site thoroughly (Fig. 6–5).
   a. Scale and root plane.
   b. Prepare a fresh incision so that the proximal gingival bed will be open with exposed connective and vascular tissues (Fig. 6–6 A,B).
   c. Expose at least 1 mm of bone and its periosteum around the defect.
2. Suture the graft into position and then hold for 2 minutes with gauze and light pressure.

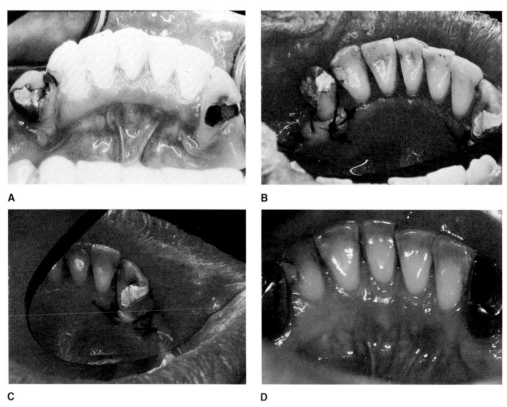

A   B

C   D

FIGURE 6–5 • Lateral pedicle graft technique. (A) Alveolar dehiscence on lingual mandibular left canine and right first premolar. The loss of tissues was caused by an ill-fitting partial denture that had settled so much that the lingual bar physically stripped the tissues away. (B) The defect area was surgically prepared to have an open vascular bed exposed around the defect, and the root was scaled and planed until smooth as glass. A pedicle flap was raised from the edentulous ridge area and placed laterally with sutures to cover the defect area. (C) The same procedure was performed on the other side. The flaps were held with gauze for 3 minutes; the area was covered with adhesive foil and then surgical dressing (Coe pack). (D) Appearance 2 years later. New crowns and new partial now cause no irritation. There is no probing depth of more than 2 mm, no bleeding on probing, and no exudates from the gingival crevices.

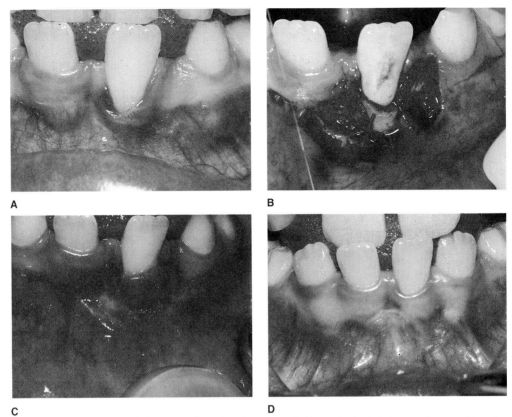

A   B

C   D

FIGURE **6–6** • Lateral pedicle gingival graft technique. (*A*) Mucogingival defect on 8-year-old male. (*B*) Tissue removed from edentulous area where lateral incisor will later erupt. Frenectomy was performed on the mesial aspect. (*C*) Appearance 1 week later. Note the revascularization of tissue. (*D*) Appearance 18 months after surgery. The lateral incisor has now erupted and has attached gingiva.

3. Cover with adhesive foil or compressed Gelfoam and the periodontal dressing.
4. Remove sutures on 5th to 7th day at first dressing change (Fig. 6–6 C).
5. Change dressings until healed (10th to 14th day).
6. Institute light physiotherapy about 30 days after surgery.
7. Do not probe forcefully for 90 days (time required for maturation of dentogingival attachments) (Fig. 6–6 D).

Free Gingival Graft

The free gingival graft is an autogenous graft of masticatory mucosa or collagenous tissue that is completely detached from its original site and blood supply and placed in a prepared recipient bed. In many cases the procedure can be used to restore gingival attachments destroyed by prostheses.

INDICATION FOR A FREE GINGIVAL GRAFT

1. Where an inadequate zone of attached gingiva is present and there is insufficient donor tissue for a lateral repositioned gingival graft (Fig. 6–7 A).

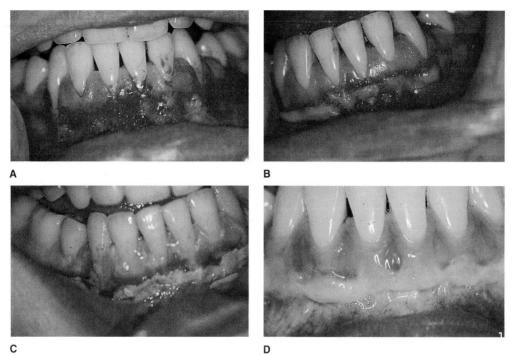

A   B

C   D

FIGURE 6–7 • Free gingival graft. (A) Alveolar dehiscences and recessions in a 20-year-old woman who had been treated orthodontically from age 12 to 15. A vascular bed is exposed apical to the recessions. (B) Gingival grafts were removed from the palate adjacent to the teeth and then placed on the exposed prepared vascular bed. Two 28-mm grafts were glued in place using cyanoacrylate at the superior junction only (not under the graft). Coe pack dressing was then placed over the wound. (C) Appearance 1 week later, after dressing was removed. Notice the white necrotic outer layer of gingival graft, which was removed with a cotton applicator and 1.5% hydrogen peroxide. A new dressing was placed for 1 more week. (D) Appearance 14 years later. Notice the graft area is whiter than the new regenerated gingiva, which is healthy and attached to the teeth. This creeping regeneration of attached gingiva occurs in many cases and can best be noted with photographic documentation.

OBJECTIVE OF THE FREE GINGIVAL GRAFT

1. To create an adequate zone of functionally attached gingiva. This is particularly important when the involved tooth will be a key abutment in an extensive restorative plan.

TECHNIQUE FOR THE FREE GINGIVAL GRAFT

1. Prepare the recipient site so that the open vascular site is ready for the graft.
2. Measure the recipient site with a probe and use this measurement when removing the donor tissue. In selecting a donor site, stay distal to the first premolar in order to stay away from rugae, and stay as close as possible to the cervical area of the teeth in order to avoid the greater palatine artery and glandular tissue.
3. Mark the epithelial side of the donor tissue with an indelible pencil. If the epithelial side is positioned against the recipient bed, the graft will fail.
4. Remove the donor tissue. Because of shrinkage, take a slightly larger than needed split-thickness donor graft (Fig. 6–7 B).

5. Hold the graft in place with gauze for 3 minutes before suturing.
6. Suture down tightly over exposed root surfaces: close coaptation of the graft to the recipient bed and tooth root is essential for success (Fig. 6–7 C,D).
7. Dress as for the lateral pedicle graft.

Figures 6–8 and 6–9 show cases in which gingival attachment was destroyed by prosthesis and repaired using the free gingival graft technique.

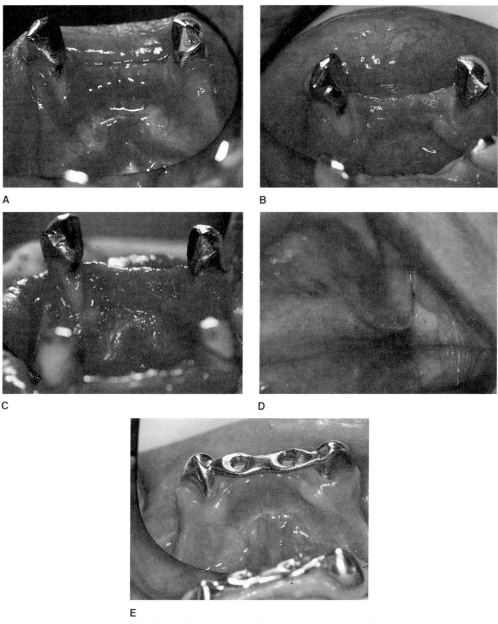

FIGURE **6–8** • Free gingival graft. (*A*) The two mandible canines are the only teeth remaining for this 45-year-old female. The lingual tissues have been destroyed by an old ill-fitting partial denture. (*B*) Edentulous ridge was chosen as the donor site. (*C*) Grafts in position over the bone. (*D*) Appearance 6 months later. Note the slight gingival regeneration on the patient's left canine above the graft. (*E*) Appearance 10 years later. Maxillary full denture and mandibular overdenture had been replaced 5 years earlier. Note the creeping reattachment on lingual.

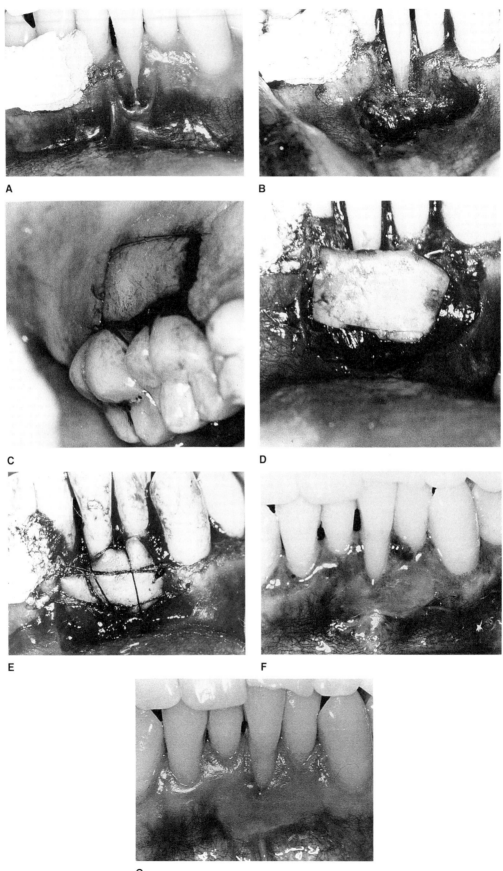

FIGURE 6–9 • Free gingival graft. (A) Mucogingival on a mandibular central incisor with no attached gingiva. (B) Receptor site prepared. (C) Donor site outlined in palate. (D) Graft coapted to receptor site. (E) Graft tightly sutured to periosteum, bone, and root. (F) Appearance at time of dressing removal. (G) Appearance 3 months later.

Free Gingival Graft for Coverage of Denuded Roots

This procedure, introduced by Dr. P. D. Miller, is similar to the free gingival graft, but more root preparation, thicker donor tissue, and use of a specialized suturing technique are required to achieve coverage of a denuded root (Fig. 6–10).

INDICATION FOR FREE GINGIVAL GRAFT FOR ROOT COVERAGE

1. Coverage of a denuded root when donor tissue for a pedicle graft is not available.

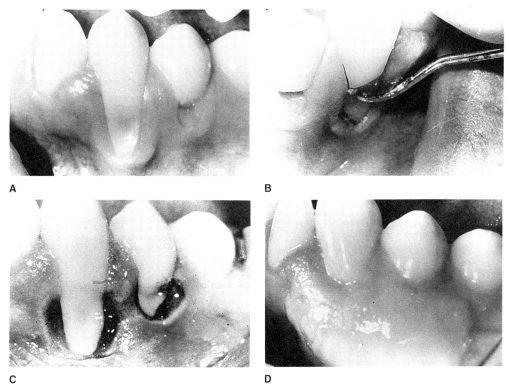

A B

C D

FIGURE 6–10 • Complete coverage of denuded roots. (A) Class II recession on an abraded mandibular canine with 7 mm of recession. (B) Root planing of the abraded, recessed area. (C) Recessed root-planed areas after 5 minutes of burnishing with citric acid. (D) Appearance 5 years later, showing complete root coverage. (Courtesy Dr. P. D. Miller)

TECHNIQUE FOR OBTAINING ROOT COVERAGE

1. Plane the root that is to receive the graft.
2. Treat with citric acid for 5 minutes.
3. Prepare recipient site with butt joints in healthy gingival tissue.
4. Remove donor tissue from palate and trim to exact fit with recipient site.
5. Suture donor tissue into recipient site so that the butt joints fit tightly together.
6. Dress as for other grafts.

In conjunction with this technique for root coverage, Dr. Miller has introduced a useful classification system for gingival recession, which is as follows:

Class I: Marginal tissue recession which does not extend to the mucogingival junction. There is no periodontal loss (bone or soft tissue) in the interdental area, and 100% root coverage can be anticipated.

Class II: Marginal tissue recession which extends to or beyond the mucogingival junction. There is no periodontal loss (bone or soft tissue) in the interdental area, and 100% root coverage can be anticipated.

Class III: Marginal tissue recession which extends to or beyond the mucogingival junction. Periodontal tissue loss is present interdentally. Partial root coverage is possible.

Class IV: Marginal tissue recession which extends beyond the mucogingival junction. Interdental tissue loss is so severe that root coverage cannot be anticipated.

Coronally Positioned Graft for Coverage of Denuded Roots

The coronally positioned graft is a pedicle graft which is moved into a coronal position in order to cover a denuded root.

INDICATION FOR CORONALLY POSITIONED GRAFT

When root coverage is desired and donor tissue is available in the immediate area.

OBJECTIVE OF THE CORONALLY POSITIONED GRAFT

To create a zone of attached gingiva covering a previously denuded root surface (Fig. 6–11 A).

TECHNIQUE FOR THE CORONALLY POSITIONED GRAFT

1. If adequate gingival tissue does not exist, place a free gingival graft apically to the exposed root as previously described (Fig. 6–11 B–D). NOTE: Vari-

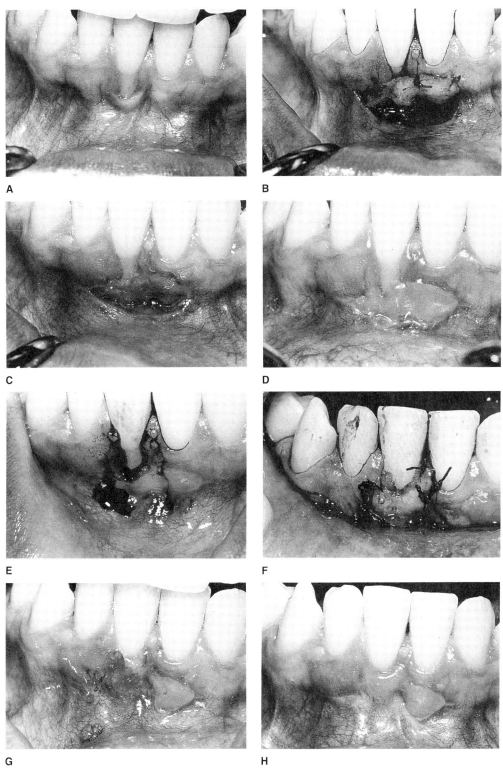

FIGURE 6–11 • Coronally positioned graft. (A) Class II recession extending to the mucogingival junction. (B) Graft placed to augment the zone of attached gingiva. (C) Appearance 1 week after surgery. (D) Appearance 8 weeks after surgery. (E) Vertical incisions through healed graft. (F) Graft sutured into coronal position. (G) Appearance 1 week after surgery. (H) Appearance 12 months after surgery. Gingiva is attached to root.

ous techniques have been published describing root coverage on previously denuded roots using the free gingival technique. Many dentists find that these procedures are not entirely reliable and frequently fail to obtain root coverage. As long as some keratinized gingiva has been placed over the periosteum apical to the denuded root, coverage can be obtained using the coronally positioned graft technique.

2. Wait approximately 8 weeks after healing of the free gingival graft before moving it coronally. This will allow adequate time for healing and revascularization.
3. Root plane the denuded root until it is glassy smooth and free of all debris.
4. Make vertical releasing incisions into the alveolar mucosa. Lift the graft and move it coronally until it is slightly higher on the tooth than you desire the final position to be. This will allow for healing retraction (Fig. 6–11 E).
5. Suture with a sling around the crown and interrupted sutures proximally (Fig. 6–11 F).
6. Hold the graft in place for 3 minutes and dress as with the lateral pedicle graft.

Conclusion

The ultimate objective of any mucogingival procedure is to restore normal anatomy and attachment. Procedures which achieve this result are technically difficult; how-

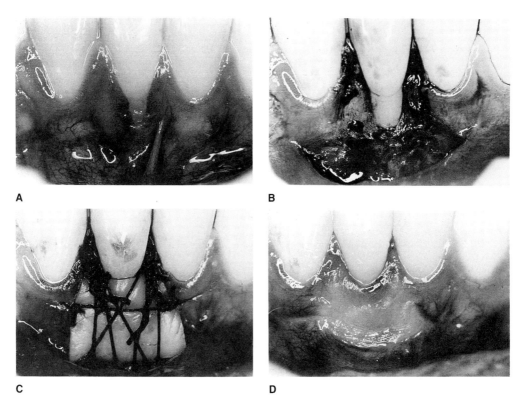

FIGURE 6–12 • Coverage of denuded roots. (A) Preoperative appearance. (B) Preparation of recipient site. (C) Graft in position. Note the precise, intricate suturing used to obtain intimate coaptation between graft and bed. (D) Initial postoperative view. Note root coverage. (Courtesy Dr. Clifford Ochsenbein)

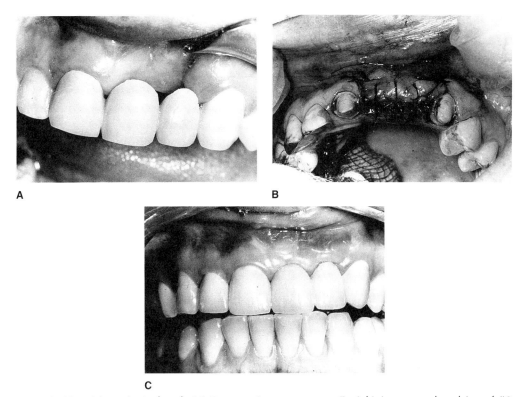

A   B

C

FIGURE 6–13 • Mucogingival graft. (A) Preoperative appearance. Facial injury caused evulsion of #9 and #10 along with a nasal-oral fistula. A provisional splint is in place after the initial accident and the nasal-oral fistula has closed. A ridge concavity remains in the area of #9 and #10. (B) A subepithelial graft from the palate has been placed in the area of #9 and #10 and the overlying flap has been sutured in place. (C) Appearance 2 months after surgery. The permanent bridge is in place. (Courtesy Dr. Burton Langer)

ever, these results are possible (Fig. 6–12). As the critical factors necessary for success with these procedures are defined, those results will become more predictable.

Frequently, extraction of periodontally diseased teeth causes functional and esthetic deficits in the alveolar ridge. Automobile accidents are another common source of damage to the alveolar ridge. Mucogingival techniques to repair such deficits are now available on a routine basis (Fig. 6–13).

Bibliography

Ammons WF Jr, Smith DH. Flap curettage: Rationale, technique and expectations. Dent Clin North Am 1976; 20:215–226.

Beaumont RH, O'Leary TJ, Kafrawy AH. Relative resistance of long junctional epithelial adhesions and connective tissue attachments to plaque-induced inflammation. J Periodontol 1984; 55:213–223.

Becker W, et al. A longitudinal study comparing scaling, osseous surgery and modified Widman procedures; Results after one year. J Periodontol 1988; 59:351–365.

Bernimoulin JP, et al. Coronally repositioned periodontal flap. J Clin Periodontol 1975; 2:1–13.

Dorfman HS, Kennedy JE, Bird WC. Longitudinal evaluation of free autologous gingival grafts. A four year report. J Periodontol 1982; 53:349–352.

Eriksson RA, Albrektsson T. The effect of heat on bone regeneration: An experimental study in the rabbit using the bone growth chamber. J Oral Maxillofac Surg 1984; 42:705–711.

Fujikawa K, O'Leary TJ, Kafrawy AH. The effect of retained subgingival calculus on healing after flap surgery. J Periodontol 1988; 59:170–175.

Gargiulo AW, Arrocha R. Histo-clinical evaluation of free gingival grafts. Periodontics 1967; 5:285–291.

Holbrook T, Ochsenbein C. Complete coverage of the denuded root surface with a one-stage gingival graft. Int J Periodont Res Dent 1983; 3:9–27.

Karn KW, et al. Topographic classification of deformities of the alveolar process. J Periodontol 1984; 55:336–340.

Kon S, et al. Revascularization following combined gingival flap: Split thickness flap procedure in monkeys. J Periodontol 1984; 55:345–351.

Langer B, and Calagna L. The subepithelial connective tissue graft. A new approach to the enhancement of anterior cosmetics. Int J Periodontics Restorative 1982: 23–29.

Litch JM, et al. Pocket epithelium removal via crestal and subcrestal scalloped internal bevel incisions. J Periodontol 1984; 55:142–148.

Miller PD. Root coverage using a free soft tissue autograft following citric acid application. Part I; technique. Int J Periodont Res Dent 1982; 2:65–70.

Morrow R. Handbook for immediate overdentures. St. Louis: CV Mosby, 1978.

Nabers J. Free gingival grafts. Periodontics 1966; 4:243–247.

Polson AM, Caton J. Factors influencing periodontal repair and regeneration. J Periodontol 1982; 53:617–625.

Svoboda PJ, et al. Effect of retention of gingival sulcular epithelium on attachment and pocket depth after periodontal surgery. J Periodontol 1984; 55:563–566.

Tenebaum H, Klewansky P, Roth JJ. Clinical evaluation of gingival recession treated by coronally repositioned flap technique. J Periodontol 1980; 51:686–690.

CHAPTER SEVEN

Treatment of Advanced Periodontitis

Patients with advanced periodontal disease (Case Type IV Code 04800—Deep pockets, severe vertical and horizontal bone loss) often require complicated treatment modalities to save their teeth. Such treatment should be initiated only when patients have a complete understanding of the severity of their problems, the prognosis for treatment, and the need for closely supervised follow-up care after treatment. Corrective therapy should not begin until patients have completed initial preparation and demonstrated their ability to control plaque.

A common finding in advanced periodontitis is advanced bone loss in one or more areas. This may be of a horizontal or a vertical nature. There are a multitude of etiologies for this condition. A retained deciduous root can cause bone loss (Fig. 7–1). Calculus on a root will also cause loss of the surrounding osseous tissue, and

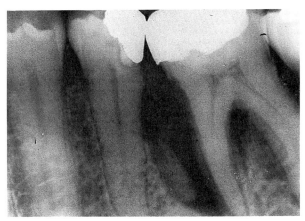

FIGURE 7–1 • Bone loss due to retained deciduous root. Note the vertical bone loss around the mesial root of the first molar. (Courtesy Dr. Bill Hurt)

101

removal of the etiologic agent will allow for repair of the bone (Fig. 7–2). A periodontal abscess will cause rapid bone loss, which can be reversed by prompt, thorough treatment (Fig. 7–3). Developmental defects in roots may contribute to bone loss. An example of this situation is the palatal groove sometimes found in maxillary lateral incisors (Fig. 7–4). Bone loss is particularly a problem in multi-rooted teeth in cases of advanced periodontitis because the furcation areas are often exposed to bacterial plaque infections. These areas cannot be cleansed so progressive bone loss often results (Fig. 7–5).

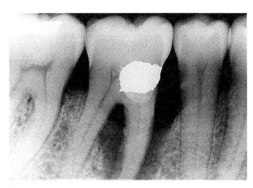 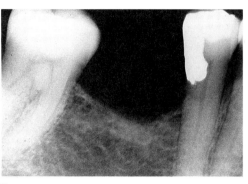

A   **B**

FIGURE 7–2 • (*A*) Bone loss due to calculus and bacterial infection of root. (*B*) Appearance 2 years after tooth was removed. There is good bone repair.

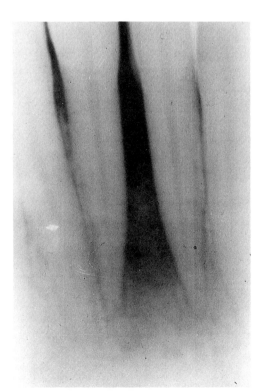 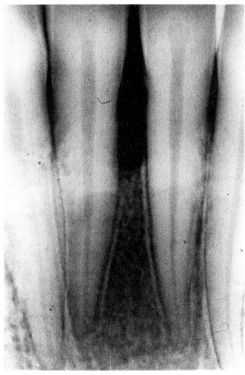

A   **B**

FIGURE 7–3 • Bone loss due to abscess. (*A*) An acute periodontal abscess has destroyed bone between the central incisors. The abscess was drained and the causative agent was removed. (*B*) Appearance 1 year later. Note bone fill. (Courtesy Dr. John Nabers)

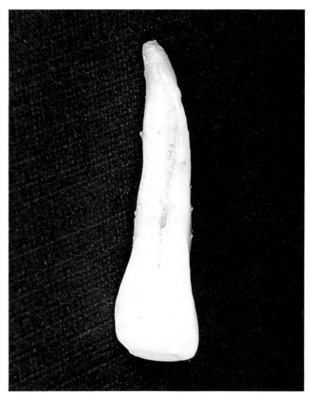

FIGURE 7–4 • Palatal groove on maxillary lateral incisor. This condition is often associated with severe bone loss.

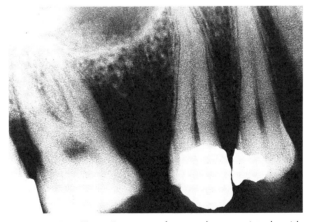

FIGURE 7–5 • Furcations are frequently associated with bone loss because they harbor bacteria once a pocket has developed.

The clinician must also look for projections of enamel into furcation areas. These make repair difficult since connective tissue will not attach to the enamel to close the defect (Figs. 7–6, 7–7). Osseous defects in anterior teeth cause special problems because of esthetic considerations (Fig. 7–8). Open contacts or placement of restorative materials which create overhangs may also cause osseous defects to develop (Fig. 7–9). Some patients develop severe osseous defects be-

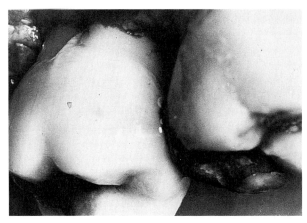

FIGURE 7–6 • Enamel projections. These are frequently associated with pockets into furcations and bone loss.

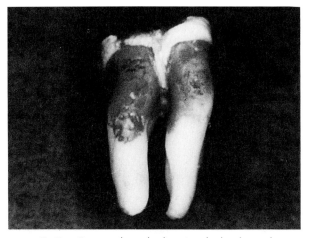

FIGURE 7–7 • Extracted tooth showing lack of attachment fibers on enamel. This lack of fibers allows faster breakdown in this area. (Courtesy Dr. Sam Hoskins)

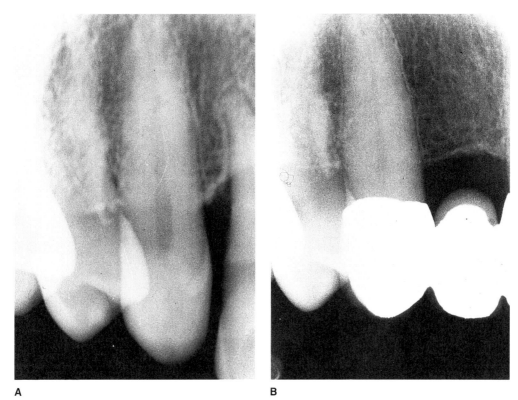

A   **B**

FIGURE 7–8 • Osseous defect in anterior teeth. (*A*) Overerupted lateral incisor with an osseous defect on the distal aspect. Because cosmetics strongly influences treatment choice in anterior teeth, the tooth was extracted and an esthetic bridge was put in place (*B*).

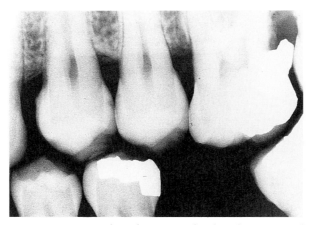

FIGURE 7–9 • Bone loss due to poorly placed contact and overhang. These defects allow plaque to build up, causing bone loss.

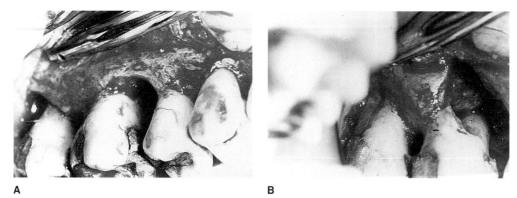

A   B

FIGURE 7–10 • Bone loss due to juvenile periodontitis. (A) Severe bone loss in a 32-year-old female. (B) Same case after mesiobuccal root was removed.

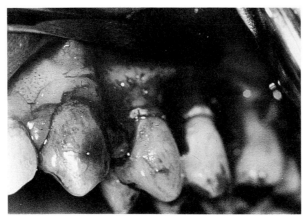

FIGURE 7–11 • Iatrogenic bone loss. Rapidly progressive bone loss was present. Orthodontic ligatures were found around the teeth when a flap was reflected.

cause of deficiences in host defense mechanisms. The most common form is juvenile periodontitis (Fig. 7–10). Iatrogenic factors may also be responsible for severe bone loss (Fig. 7–11).

Bone Fill Surgery

Bone fill surgery is a surgical procedure designed to stimulate bone repair without the use of graft materials.

INDICATIONS FOR BONE FILL SURGERY

1. Bone destruction following any acute abscess. (Inform the patient that in 6 months a secondary operation may be needed to contour bone and eliminate soft-tissue pocketing.)

2. Thin three-wall osseous defects. These are defects surrounded by bone on three sides. They have a good prognosis with bone fill (Fig. 7–12).
3. One- and two-wall osseous defects where regeneration therapy is not indicated and the tooth or teeth involved have a guarded prognosis. (Such areas often require retreatment in 4 to 6 years.)

OBJECTIVES OF BONE FILL SURGERY

1. To obtain as much bone fill as possible for the indications shown above.
2. To maintain teeth without jeopardizing adjacent teeth.

TECHNIQUE FOR BONE FILL SURGERY

1. Use a full flap for access and retain as much interproximal gingiva as possible to facilitate complete closure.
2. Perform thorough scaling and root planing.
3. Remove all soft tissue from the osseous defect.
4. Cut small holes with a small round bur through any dense sclerotic bone lining the defect to the adjacent vascular medullary spaces. This improves the potential for revascularization in the osseous defect area.

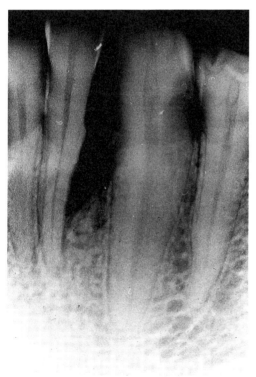 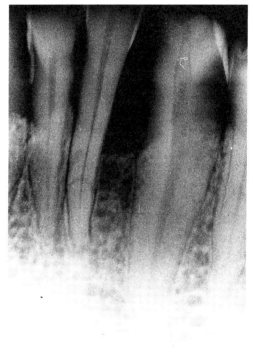

A   **B**

FIGURE 7–12 • Three-wall osseous defect. (*A*) Preoperative appearance. (*B*) Appearance 1 year after bone fill surgery.

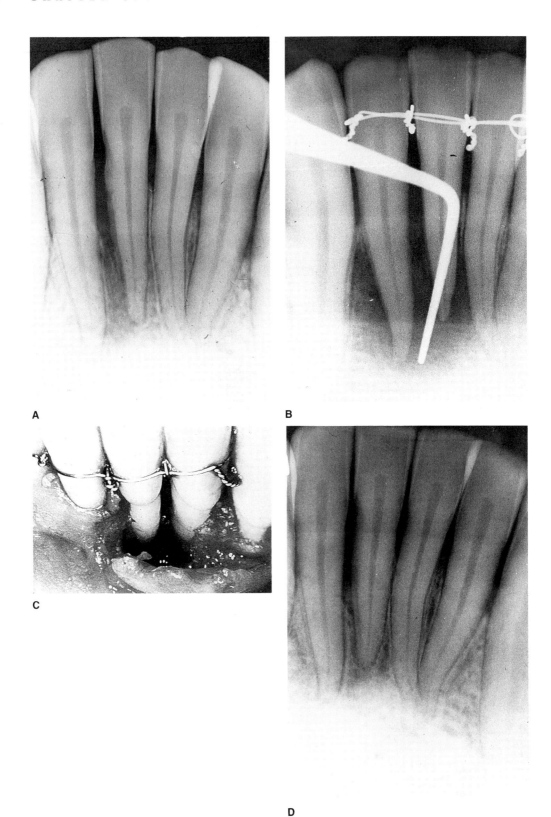

FIGURE 7–13 • Bone fill surgery. (*A*) Radiographic appearance at initial examination. (*B*) Appearance a few days later. Note bone loss. Patient had an acute abscess and the teeth were loose. Systemic antibiotic therapy was initiated and the teeth were ligated with orthodontic ligature wires. Sometimes probing or partial scaling can cause an acute abscess. (*C*) Appearance at time of bone fill operation. Notice the hole, which extended to the apices of the teeth. (*D*) Appearance 5 months later. Bone height is back to about pre-abscess level.

5. Remove any inflammatory tissue or epithelium from within the gingival flap so that an open vascular surface covers the osseous defect (Fig. 7–13).
6. Coapt the area completely by suturing.
7. If the osseous defect is so large that the flap falls into it, place a membrane over in the hole as a scaffold for the gingiva, using the technique described for the guided tissue regeneration procedure later in this chapter.

Prichard's Intrabony Procedure

Prichard's intrabony procedure is a surgical procedure designed to accomplish bone repair in intrabony defects.

INDICATION FOR THE INTRABONY PROCEDURE

To repair intrabony defects.

OBJECTIVE OF THE INTRABONY PROCEDURE

To obtain deposition of cementum, bone, and a new connective tissue attachment to the tooth (Fig. 7–14).

TECHNIQUE FOR THE INTRABONY PROCEDURE

1. Remove the gingiva to the coronal margins of the bony defect.
2. Remove all granulation tissue and periodontal ligament fibers from the defect. (Use curettes, not burs.)
3. Remove all calculus from the root but leave cementum.
4. Cover the osseous defects and teeth with foil to keep surgical dressing out.
5. Use antibiotics for 1 week after surgery.
6. Adjust occlusion if tooth is in trauma.

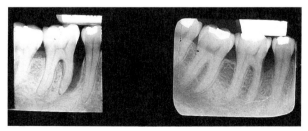

FIGURE **7–14** • Prichard's intrabony technique. (*Left*) Intrabony defect. (*Right*) Same area 8 years after treatment. (Courtesy Dr. John Prichard)

Additional considerations for the intrabony procedure

1. Presurgical scaling is not done with this technique. Removal of calculus is accomplished at the time of surgery. Many periodontists feel that this provides a greater stimulus to healing.
2. Success with this technique has not been reported in teeth which had received endodontic filling before surgery.
3. Care must be taken to ensure that soft tissues are not closed over the defect, as this will allow epithelium to proliferate into the defect first.
4. Because bone tissue is left exposed, the postoperative course can be more painful.

Guided Tissue Regeneration

Guided tissue regeneration (GTR) is a surgical procedure designed to guide healing of the surgical wound in such a manner that repair is by new attachment.

Indication for GTR

1. To restore periodontal attachment in furcation involvements and vertical defects.

Objective of GTR

1. To restore lost connective tissue attachment to the root surface by excluding the epithelium long enough to allow connective tissue to repopulate the wound.

Technique for GTR

1. Make intrasulcular incisions to preserve as much tissue in the flap as possible. Expose the defect completely so that it can be thoroughly debrided and epithelial blocking material can be placed (Figs. 7–15 A, 7–15 B). (Millipore filters were used in the original research for this purpose.)
2. Remove all granulation tissue and thoroughly scale the root surface.
3. Form blocking material to go from the bone to the tooth and suture the material either to the inside of the flap or around the tooth itself. Use a slow-resorbing suture such as Dexon for this (Fig. 7–15 C). (The W. F. Gore Company currently makes a material designed specifically for this procedure which has an open microstructure collar that inhibits epithelial downgrowth.)
4. After the material is placed over the bone to cover the defect, suture the flaps to completely cover the material if possible.

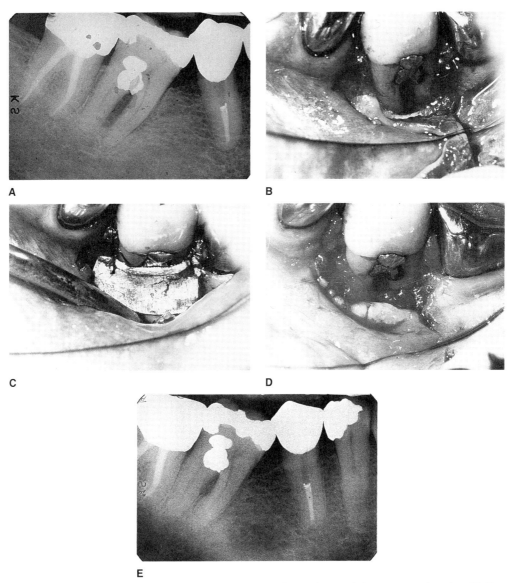

FIGURE 7–15 • Guided tissue regeneration. (*A*) Deep Class II furcae defect in second molar. (*B*) Defect exposed and debrided. (*C*) Sterile membrane placed over the exposed furca to block out the epithelium. (*D*) Same area 1 month later at the time of membrane removal. Note healing of connective tissue coronal on roots and furca. (*E*) Same area as in *A* 18 months after surgery. Note new osseous tissue in furca.

5. Leave the material in place for 1 to 3 months and then remove it during a secondary procedure (Fig. 7–15 D). Do not root plane the tooth during the secondary procedure as you will remove the newly formed periodontal ligament. Curette the inside of the flap lightly to remove epithelium.

Do not expect bone to regenerate with this technique. If case selection has been proper and the procedure is performed correctly, however, you may expect new connective tissue attachment to the previously diseased root. This will stop attachment loss and preserve the tooth (Fig. 7–15 E).

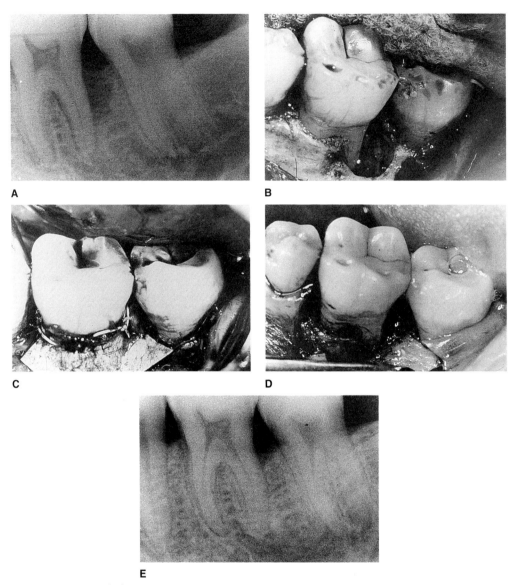

FIGURE 7–16 • Guided tissue regeneration. (*A*) Preoperative radiograph of an osseous defect distal to the mandibular first molar. (*B*) Preoperative view of deep intrabony defect after cleaning of the roots and bone. (*C*) Gore-tex periodontal membrane in place over the defect. (*D*) Area re-entered at 11 months. Note complete regeneration. The material had been removed at 30 days. (*E*) Radiograph showing bone regeneration 11 months after surgery. (Courtesy Drs. William and Burton Becker)

Bone Grafting

Bone grafting is the process of repairing bony defects by means of autografts, allografts, or alloplasts. It requires a healthy patient who has a strong desire to keep his own teeth and who has demonstrated his effectiveness in performing oral hygiene.

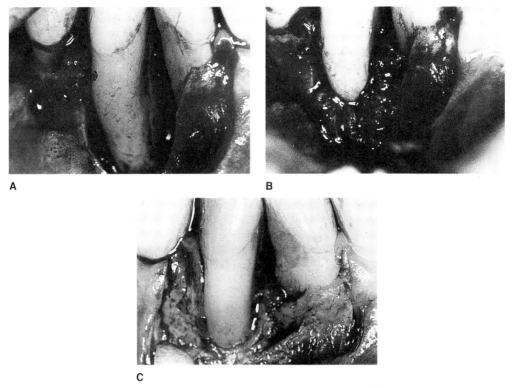

FIGURE 7–17 • Autogenous bone grafting. (*A*) Exposed defect on mandibular canine. (*B*) Autogenous bone from maxilla placed in defect. (*C*) Same area at re-entry. Note bone fill. (Courtesy Drs. Marvin, Edward, and Richard Sugarman)

AUTOGENOUS BONE GRAFT (ABG)

An autogenous bone graft, or autograft, is a graft taken from the patient's own body. There are many donor sites available when doing autogenous bone grafts. The materials used include bone chips (shavings from osteoplasty and ostectomy) and cancellous material from the posterior maxilla (Fig. 7–17). Immature bone from a healing extraction site has good regeneration potential when it can be obtained (Fig. 7–18). Osseous coagulum is defined as small bone particles obtained from grinding which are mixed with the patient's blood then placed into the defects. Cancellous red marrow has been reported to give the greatest amount of bone fill. It is often impractical, however, to secure bone from the iliac crest for use in the dental office. Furthermore, this material must be frozen before use to decrease the possibility of root resorption.

ALLOGRAFTS

If sufficient autogenous material cannot be secured, an allograft may be used as the donor material. Many tissue banks currently sell this material. Although its osteogenic potential does not seem to be as great as that of autogenous bone, allograft material is better than an alloplastic material or no graft at all. Freeze-dried decalcified bone has more osteogenic potential than freeze-dried bone that has not been decalcified.

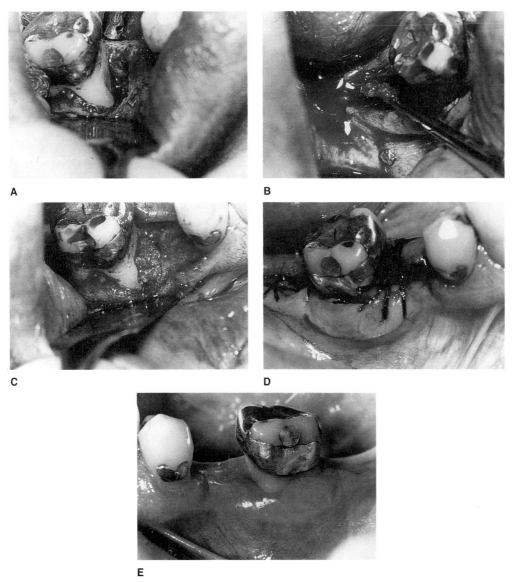

FIGURE 7–18 • Autogenous bone grafts. (*A*) Defect on mesial first molar. (*B*) Healing osteoid taken from extraction socket where second molar had been removed 12 weeks before. (*C*) Graft placed in osseous defect mesial to molar. (*D*) Area sutured with primary closure. (*E*) Appearance 3 months after surgery (mirror view). Area could not be probed more than 3 mm.

ALLOPLASTS

These materials are a substitute for autogenous bone. In our opinion, however, the clinician will obtain a better long-term result with autogenous bone grafts.

The currently available alloplastic materials are tricalcium phosphate, which is partially resorbable, and hydroxylapatite, which is non-resorbable.

Controlled studies have shown that implantation of tricalcium phosphate tends to produce better pocket closure and slower regression than debridement alone. However, histologic observations have not demonstrated any new connective tissue attachment resulting from the use of this material.

Studies using hydroxylapatite have shown that it, too, yields a greater reduction in pocket depth in bony defects than treatment with debridement alone. New attachment has not been demonstrated with this material either.

INDICATIONS FOR BONE GRAFTS

1. Osseous defect in which bone fill is not likely without a bone graft.
2. Osseous defect that has only one or two walls, but has retaining contours to hold the graft in place.
3. Good prognosis on the involved tooth if the bone graft is successful.

OBJECTIVES OF BONE GRAFTS

1. To obtain bone repair in an osseous defect. Success depends on proper development of the healing cells.
2. To save isolated teeth that are important to an arch.

TECHNIQUE FOR BONE GRAFTS

1. Expose the osseous defect by a flap approach saving the interdental papilla and all the gingiva possible so that complete coverage over the graft can be accomplished when sutured at the finish of the surgery (Fig. 7–19 A).

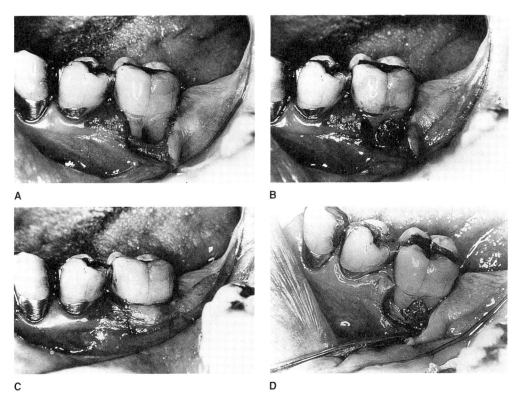

A   B

C   D

FIGURE 7–19 • Autogenous bone graft. (A) Class III furca on mandibular molar. (B) Iliac crest marrow placed in the defect. (C) Primary closure. (D) Re-entry at 5 months. Note bone fill in the furca. (Courtesy Dr. Robert Schallhorn)

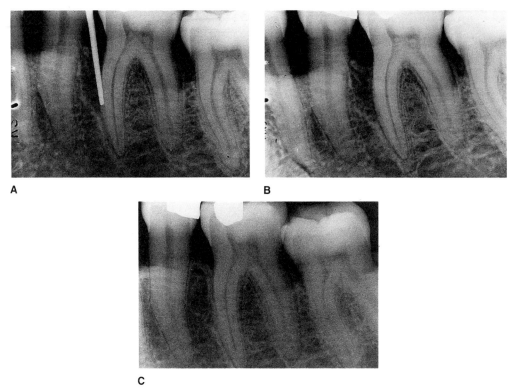

FIGURE 7–20 • Autogenous bone graft. (*A*) Bony defect with probe in place. (*B*) Radiograph taken immediately after surgery showing bone particles in place. (*C*) Radiograph taken 24 years later. Note complete fill of the defect.

2. Prepare the osseous defect and root as for bone fill surgery.
3. Cut small bur holes through the sclerotic bone of the defect area to help vascularize area for healing.
4. Thoroughly plane roots adjacent to the defect.
5. Obtain graft material from the donor site and place it into the defect so that it is completely filled (Fig. 7–19 B).
6. Use systemic antibiotic coverage for 1 week after surgery.
7. Obtain primary flap closure (Fig. 7–19 C).
8. Pay close attention to the involved area while healing is in progress. Remove all plaque and deposits with instrumentation at each visit every 2 weeks for 3 months.
9. To see how the graft is progressing, x-ray the area at 3- to 4-month intervals for 1 year (Fig. 7–20).

Combined Endodontic and Periodontal Therapy

When a tooth has a combined endodontic and a periodontal involvement one must first make a differential diagnosis of periodontal and pulpal pathosis. If an apparent periodontal abscess occurs in a bifurcation or trifurcation, or approaches the apical third of an involved root, it is extremely important to rule out pulpal pathosis. Pulpal pathosis can be determined by lack of vitality or by the presence of a sinus tract.

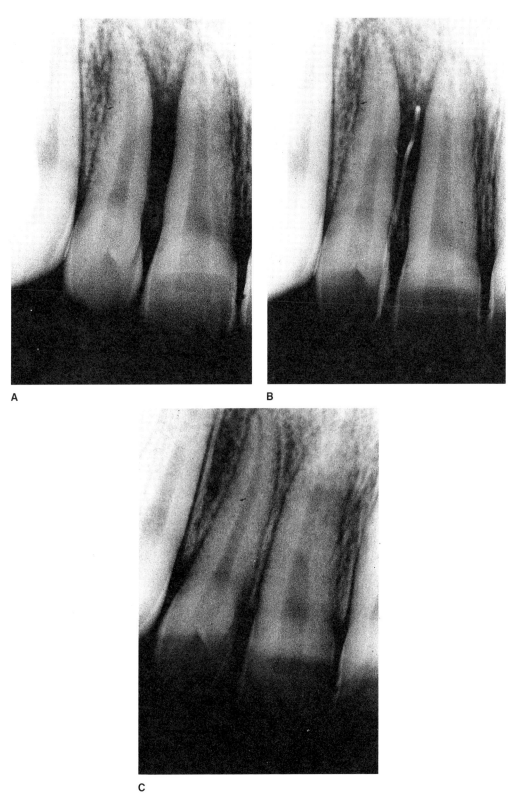

FIGURE **7–21** • Exploration of a fistulous tract. (*A*) An abscess between the central and lateral incisors. (*B*) Gutta-percha probe exploring the source of the defect. (*C*) Appearance after periodontal therapy. There is complete regeneration of bone. The patient was originally referred for endodontics. (Courtesy Dr. Hub Lundblade)

Test the vitality of the teeth in the involved area. A symptomatic devital tooth will require endodontic treatment or extraction. If a fistulous tract is present, place gutta-percha into it until resistance is met; x-ray it with the gutta-percha point in place. The film may show the point to be at the apex of one of the teeth, indicating pulpal pathosis (Fig. 7–21).

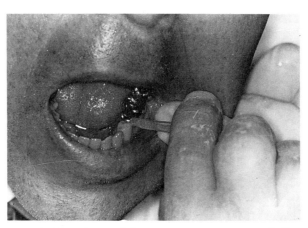

FIGURE 7–22 • Ice on full coverage crown to test vitality. An ice rod can easily be made in a used anesthetic carpule.

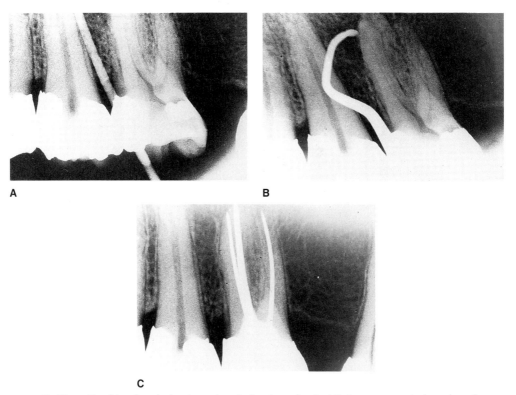

FIGURE 7–23 • Combined endodontic and periodontic pathosis. (A) Apparent periodontal pocket on the mesial aspect of the second molar. A gutta-percha point is in the pocket. (B) Appearance at the time of an exploratory operation which revealed the source of the problem to be at the apex of the first molar. Note the instrument going through the defect to the apex of the adjoining tooth. (C) Appearance after completion of the endodontic treatment on the first molar. There was complete regeneration of the destroyed bone on the second molar. No periodontal therapy was required. (Courtesy Dr. Hub Lundblade)

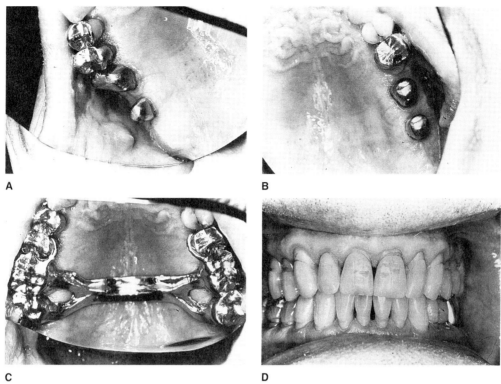

A   B   C   D

FIGURE 7–24 • Root amputation. (*A*) Lingual root of the second molar was retained with endodontic treatment and a short coping crown. Distobuccal root of the first molar was amputated after endodontic therapy. (*B*) Lingual roots were retained on the first and second molars with endodontic treatment and short coping crowns. (*C*) Tooth-supported precision attachment partial denture is supported by retained roots of molars. (*D*) Appearance 8 years after surgery. No clasps show.

If crowns are on the teeth, it may be necessary to test the crowned tooth or teeth with ice or dry ice, or even drill a test hole through the crown with no local anesthesia to bur-test the dentin for vitality (Fig. 7-22). When endodontic therapy is indicated, it should be initiated as soon as possible. When your examination of the data indicates the presence of both pulpal pathosis and untreatable advanced periodontal involvement, then suggest extraction of the involved tooth after therapeutic blood levels of antibiotic are obtained. (This can be as little as 2 hours after antibiotics are started.)

If pulpal pathosis has established drainage through the periodontium simulating a periodontal pocket, initiate endodontic therapy and wait for healing before treating the pseudoperiodontal pocket (Fig. 7–23).

Initiate endodontic and periodontic treatment if pulpal pathosis is combined with a treatable periodontal pocket associated with an acute periodontal abscess or a thin three-wall defect.

Endodontics and Root Amputations

There are times when a multiple-rooted tooth is needed for a bridge abutment or to improve the prognosis of an arch. If the periodontal pathosis involves one root of the tooth only, consider amputation of that one root after endodontic therapy on the tooth. Also to be considered is the possibility of saving part of a tooth to be used as a support for a partial or full denture (Fig. 7–24).

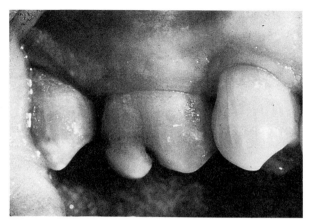

FIGURE 7–25 • Maxillary first molar in linguoversion with Class III furcal involvements from the mesial. Palatal root was amputated. (Courtesy Dr. Donald Newell)

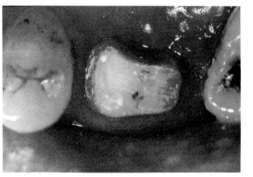
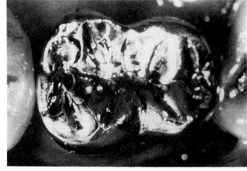

A   B

FIGURE 7–26 • (A) Buccal roots of tooth in Fig. 7–25 prepared for crown. (Courtesy Dr. Eugene Appleton). (B) Buccal roots restored with crown that fits within contours of the arch. (Courtesy Dr. Donald Newell)

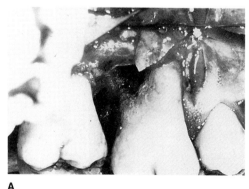
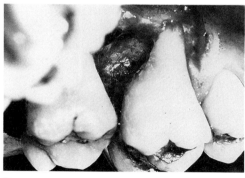

A   B

FIGURE 7–27 • Root amputation. (A) First molar exposed. Area had been treated with a distobuccal root amputation 1 year before. However, a portion of the root was not removed, and inflammation and pocket depth persisted. (B) Root has been contoured to remove all of the distobuccal root and contour the furca into the crown area.

When root amputation is performed, the apical portion of that part of the crown must be contoured to blend smoothly with the remaining roots (Figs. 7–25, 7–26).

Chronic inflammation and pockets will remain if portions of the amputated root are left behind. Good surgical access and careful instrumentation are necessary to accomplish this difficult procedure properly (Fig. 7–27).

When mandibular molars are resected it is often necessary to move the attached gingiva from the ridge mesially or distally to close the extraction site of the removed root (Fig. 7–28 A–G).

In maxillary molars it is often necessary to resect a root in order to eliminate a furcation or allow for more interproximal bone (Figures 7–29 A–C).

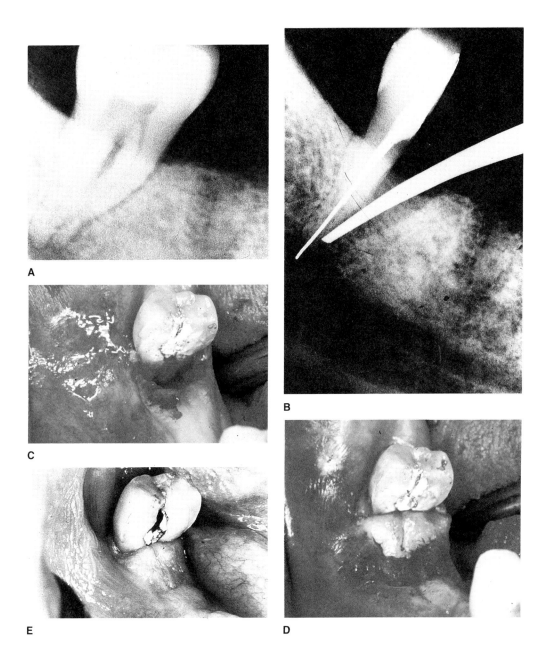

A

B

C

E

D

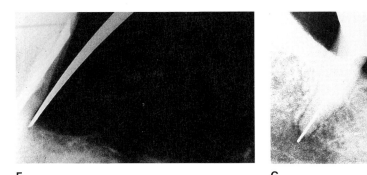

F   **G**

FIGURE 7–28 • Root amputation in mandibular molar. (A) Preoperative appearance. There is deep furcation involvement on the second molar. The first molar is missing. (B) Appearance after endodontics and mesial root amputation. Radiograph shows chisel being used to root plane. (C) Clinical view of the area after hemisection of the mesial root. (D) Hiatt's ridge flap graft has been moved distally to completely cover the defect. Buccal and lingual blood supplies are retained to nourish the graft. (E) Appearance 4 months after surgery. (F) Thin instrument used to vigorously probe area. (G) Radiographic appearance 22 years after surgery. (Courtesy Dr. William Hiatt)

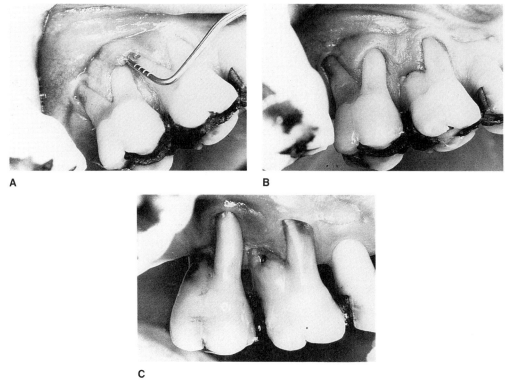

A   **B**

C

FIGURE 7–29 • Root amputation in maxillary molar. (A) A periodontal abscess has occurred as a result of the convergence of the molar roots and the lack of interdental tissue. (B) Removal of the distobuccal root after endodontic therapy and a retrograde alloy, shows the healed area five years later. (C) Appearance 25 years later. (The distobuccal root of the second molar had been removed 15 years previously.) The interdental area remains free of disease. (Courtesy Dr. Gerald Kramer)

Bibliography

Amen CR. Hemisection and root amputation. Periodontics 1966; 4:197–204.

Baldock WT, Hutchens LH Jr, McFall WT, Simpson DM. An evaluation of tricalcium phosphate implants in human periodontal osseous defects of two patients. J Periodontol 1985; 56:1–7.

Bühler H. Evaluation of root resected teeth. J Periodontol 1988; 59:805–810.

Ellegaard B. Bone grafts in periodontal attachment procedures. J Clin Periodontol 1976; 3(5):1–54.

Gleckner JG, Hurt WC. Case reports. Retained deciduous root tips and intrabony pocket formation. Armed Forces Med J 1960; 11:1049–1051.

Goldman HM, Scholder H. Regeneration of attachment apparatus lost due to disease of endodontic origin. J. Periodontol 1988; 59:609–610.

Gottlow J, Nyman S, Karring T, Lindhe J. New attachment formation as a result of controlled tissue regeneration. J Clin Periodontol 1984; 11:494–503.

Gottlow J, Nyman S, Lindhe J, Karring T, Wennstrom J. New attachment formation in the human periodontium by guided tissue regeneration. J Clin Periodontol 1986; 13:604–616.

Hellden LB, et al. The prognosis of tunnel preparations in treatment of class III furcations. A follow-up study. J. Periodontol 1989; 60:182–187.

Hiatt WH. Periodontal pocket elimination by combined endodontic-periodontic therapy. J Periodontol 1963; 1:152–159.

Magnusson I, et al. New attachment formation following controlled tissue regeneration using biodegradable membranes. J Periodontol 1988; 59:1–6.

Marinak KW. The osteogenic potential of two human demineralized bone preparations using a xenogeneic model. J Periodontol 1989; 60:12–18.

Masters D, Hoskins S. Projections of cervical enamel in molar furcations. J Periodontol 1964; 35:49–53.

Mattout P, Roche M. Juvenile periodontitis: Healing following autogenous iliac marrow graft, long-term evaluation. J Clin Periodontol 1984; 11:274–279.

McHugh WD. The effects of exclusion of epithelium from healing periodontal pockets. J Periodontol 1988; 59:750–757.

Meffert RM, et al. Hydroxylapatite as an alloplastic graft in the treatment of human periodontal osseous defects. J Periodontol 1985; 56:63–73.

Mellonig JT. Alveolar bone induction: Autografts and allografts. Dent Clin North Am 1980; 719–737.

Movin S, Borring-Moller G. Regeneration of infrabony periodontal defects in humans after implantation of allogenic demineralized dentin. J. Clin Periodontol 1982; 9:141–147.

Nabers CL. Long-term results of autogenous bone grafts. Int J Periodont Restorative Dent 1984; 3:51–67.

Nabers CL, et al. In order to secure "fill" in osseous defects is it necessary or desirable to "plane" the exposed root surfaces until they are hard and smooth to the touch? J Periodontol 1970; 41:419–423.

O'Leary TJ, et al. Periodontal therapy: A summary status report 1987–1988. J Periodontol 1988; 59:306–310.

Prichard JF. The diagnosis and management of vertical bony defects. J Periodontol 1983; 54:29–35.

Quattlebaum JB, et al. Antigenicity of freeze-dried cortical bone allograft in human periodontal osseous defects. J Periodontol 1988; 59:394–397.

Register AA, Burdick FA. Accelerated reattachment with cementogenesis to dentin, demineralized in situ. J Periodontol 1976; 47(9):497–505.

Robinson RE. Osseous coagulum for bone induction. J Periodontol 1969; 40:503–510.

Schallhorn RG. The use of autogenous hip marrow biopsy implants for bony crater defects. J Periodontol 1968; 39:145–147.

Soehren SE, Van Swol RL. The healing extraction site: A donor area for periodontal grafting material. J Periodontol 1979; 50(3):128–133.

Stahl SS, Froum S. Histological evaluation of human intraosseous healing responses to the placement of tricalcium phosphate ceramic implants. I. Three to eight months. J Periodontol 1986; 57(4):211–217.

Tanner MG, et al. An evaluation of new attachment formation using a microfibrillar collagen barrier. J Periodontol 1988; 59:524–530.

CHAPTER EIGHT

Supportive Therapies

Occlusion

The study of occlusion is a complex and difficult phase of dentistry. There are several biological considerations to keep in mind when occlusion is to be considered. Teeth are not in a static position. With attritional occlusal wear, passive continuous eruption compensates for the wear. Also, to compensate for the proximal wear at the contacts, there is mesial drift. In one sense this is good, for there is a constant turnover of the living cells forming the periodontal ligaments, cementum, and bone. A second biological consideration to keep in mind is that when teeth are moved in any direction by applied forces, they do not return to their original positions but only partially recover.*

Most schools of thought on occlusion agree that a mutually protected occlusion is best. This means that when patients interdigitate in centric position the posterior teeth contact, and when lateral or protrusive movements of the mandible are made there will be a disclusion of the posterior teeth with occlusal contacts on the canines and on anterior teeth. Because of myofunctional habits such as tongue thrusting, some people can only occlude their most posterior teeth. If myofunctional therapy is instituted promptly—and ideally early in life—patients can establish a healthier occlusion. If such patients are treated orthodontically a good result can be obtained, but if myofunctional therapy is not properly followed the ultimate result will usually be the same as before orthodontics. Likewise, all orthodontic results should be accomplished in such a way that the patient's centric relation, centric occlusion, and eccentric movements are correlated to the function of the temporomandibular joints and the muscles of mastication. Remember to look for deviations of the nose and the nasal septum as well as lack of symmetry of maxilla, mandible, and cheeks. These are often the result of sleeping mainly on one side or

---

*To study lateral movement of teeth most mobilometer studies apply 500 grams of force to the lingual and then to the buccal aspects of a tooth. The mobility of the tooth is then measured from its most buccal to its most lingual position. Under these stresses the tooth does not return to the central or neutral position.

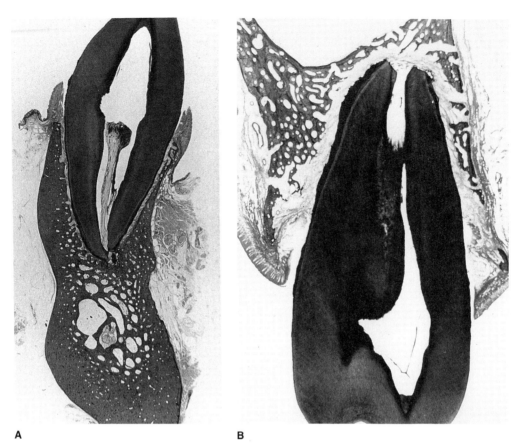

A   **B**

FIGURE **8–1** • Effect of occlusal trauma. (A) Thin, uniform periodontal ligament space in this nec-ropsy section indicates a lack of occlusal trauma and normal functional adaptation. (B) Widened periodontal ligament in this necropsy section of a maxillary molar indicates that the connective tissues were accommodating for excess occlusal pressure.

on a hand. These habits are hard to change. Such sleeping patterns can also create centric prematurities.

Occlusion Adjustment

Whereas it was previously believed that occlusal trauma contributed significantly to the etiology of periodontitis, controlled studies in animals have indicated that oc-clusal trauma in the absence of inflammation will not result in attachment loss. However, these studies have also shown that attachment loss is greater and less amenable to repair where occlusal trauma is superimposed on a tooth or teeth with inflamed periodontal tissues. Of course, data from animal studies are not reliably transferable to humans, so treatment of the occlusion as part of periodontal therapy remains controversial. Since inflammation is usually not completely eliminated in patients, it is advisable for the therapist to eliminate major occlusal discrepancies in order to obtain the best result possible. Widened periodontal ligaments are more susceptible to periodontal breakdown (Fig. 8–1 B).

Treatment of occlusal discrepancies can be incorporated at various times dur-ing the overall therapy. We usually plan to adjust the occlusion, when indicated, while waiting for anesthesia for scaling, curettage, or surgery, and at finish appoint-ments. The bilateral manipulation technique is used to determine centric relation

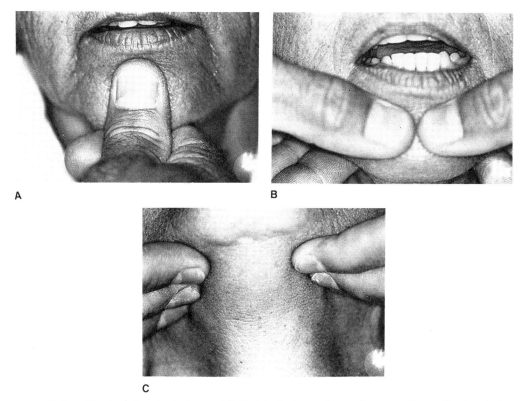

FIGURE 8–2 • Manipulation techniques. (A) Old technique of retruding mandible with thumb for centric relation. (B) Dawson technique. Thumbs are positioned on chin for the start of Dr. Peter Dawson's technique of bilateral manipulation to precisely determine the centric relation. This can be accurately reproduced. (C) With the Dawson technique, finger tips are placed on the inferior border of the mandible with an upper pressure to seat the condyles in their uppermost (apex of force) position. Note pressure causes blanching of fingernails. This technique will usually eliminate muscle spasms and temporomandibular joint pain if the mandible is manipulated for 2 to 3 minutes.

and functional excursions (Figure 8–2). Figure 8–3 demonstrates the importance of checking the occlusion in function. The danger of creating a positive occlusal sense is lessened if occlusal changes are accomplished while the patient's mouth is anesthetized.* One must remember that the occlusal relationships are dynamic in that they are constantly changing and should be continuously monitored.

INDICATIONS FOR OCCLUSAL ADJUSTMENT

1. Slight prematurity in centric relationship on a mobile tooth.
2. Balance-side discrepancy in lateral excursions with possible wandering of maxillary anterior teeth.
3. Chipped sharp edges on teeth.
4. Lack of cosmetic harmony in anterior teeth.
5. Mobility of one tooth with adequate bone support.
6. Lack of protrusive balance in anterior teeth.

---

*"Positive occlusal sense" is a condition in which the patient is constantly aware of the way that the teeth come together and is looking for problems in the occlusion. If you cannot find physiological evidence of occlusal discrepancy you should suspect a psychological component and avoid intervention.

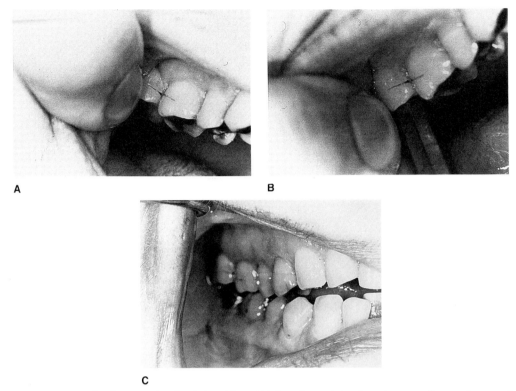

A   B

C

FIGURE 8–3 • Checking occlusal relationships. (*A*) Pencil mark is placed across first and second molar to identify their relationship to each other. (*B*) Pressure exerted on second molar with a mirror handle shows no depression. (*C*) When patient bites hard in centric relation, second molar is depressed. (Courtesy Dr. James O'Bannon)

OBJECTIVES OF OCCLUSAL ADJUSTMENT

1. To create an occlusion that is in harmony with the temporomandibular joints and muscles of mastication so that when the mandible is closed from its relaxed posterior resting position the teeth interdigitate evenly and in unison.
2. To obtain harmony for the working side on lateral excursions and avoid interferences or tripping on the balance side. Anterior disclusion or anterior guidance is always desired, when possible, to help protect the posterior teeth.
3. To create prettier teeth, when possible, and to eliminate the possibility of trauma to the tongue or lips from chipped teeth with jagged or saw-toothed edges.
4. To eliminate excessive or lateral stresses on a tooth with primary occlusal traumatism.

NOTE: One must be careful in occlusal adjustments not to create a positive occlusal sense in a patient that will transform him into a dental neurotic or dental psychotic. If there is not a clear indication for occlusal adjustment, do nothing. Also, remember that occlusal adjustments alone will not cure moderate-to-advanced occlusal disharmonies, which may require orthognathic surgery or occlusal reconstruction. Occlusal discrepancies may occur with all degrees of periodontal disease, but they are not considered a major complication in gingivitis unless there is a concurrent myofascial pain dysfunction syndrome.

TECHNIQUE FOR OCCLUSAL ADJUSTMENT

1. Using the bilateral manipulation technique, position the mandible into centric relation while your assistant holds a thin silk typewriter ribbon between the patient's teeth. The ribbon is then removed and the teeth are tapped lightly together with nothing between them. This will create a halo (white center within the mark) that indicates precisely which areas do in fact contact (Fig. 8–4 A).
2. Remove prematurities and contact areas on inclined planes.
3. Continue this process until halos are on cusp tips and marginal ridges, centric relation coincides with centric occlusion, and the patient's bite is even and comfortable (Fig. 8–4 B).
4. Test for contacts between natural and prosthetic teeth (Fig. 8–5). (We often use thin shimstock [5/10,000-inch thickness] for this purpose.)
5. Check for balancing or non-working interferences. This is important, as these may contribute to temporomandibular joint or periodontal problems (Fig. 8–6).

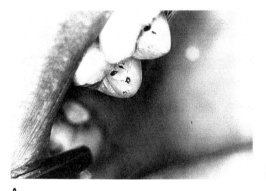
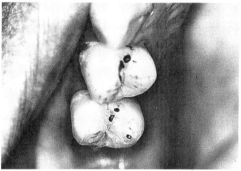

A   **B**

FIGURE **8–4** • Technique for occlusal adjustment. (A) Marking of contact areas. Notice the halos on the second premolar are on inclined planes. High-speed diamonds are used to polish off the halos. They are then rechecked and polished further. (B) Adjustment completed. Note positions of halos.

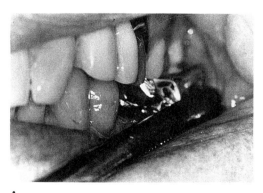
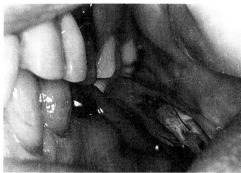

A   **B**

FIGURE **8–5** • Checking occlusal contact. (A) Light pressure by patient prevents the shimstock from sliding out. (B) Thin shimstock being used to test occlusal contacts of a partial denture.

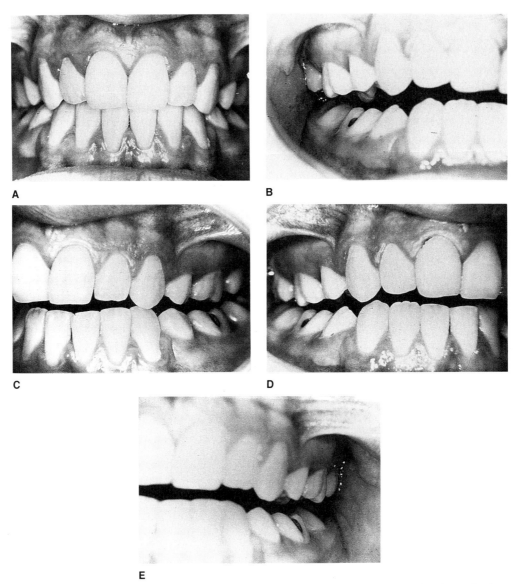

A

B

C

D

E

FIGURE 8–6 • Checking for balancing interferences. (A) Centric occlusion 18 months after orthodontic treatment. Occlusal contact is good but patient has temporomandibular joint pain. (B) Left working relationship. There is a balancing contact on the right side. (C) Left working relationship. (D) Right working relationship. Patient cannot touch teeth except in second molar area. (E) Severe left balancing contact keeping teeth apart during right working relationship. (Courtesy Dr. Jay S. Seibert)

CONTRAINDICATIONS FOR OCCLUSAL ADJUSTMENTS

Occlusal adjustment should not be done when all the patient's teeth are worn flat and display centric prematurity, nonfunctional interferences, or lack of anterior guidance.

Arch discrepancies such as a broad maxilla and a narrow mandible with the patient functioning in an acquired centric relationship also constitute contraindications. These cases are an indication for orthodontic correction, surgical correction, or a combination of the two.

Occlusal adjustment should not be done when there is a gross discrepancy between centric relation and centric occlusion. In this type of case mount duplicate models on an articulator and perform occlusal adjustments on the models to determine if the end result corrects the occlusal discrepancies, or if it might create a bigger problem than the one that is present in the beginning.

Occlusion adjustment is also contraindicated when all the teeth are mobile because of secondary occlusal trauma (i.e., mobility due to advanced loss of support for the teeth). In such cases the teeth may need to be stabilized before corrective surgery is performed.

A patient with a positive occlusal sense who has previously had occlusal adjustments by other doctors should not be adjusted. This patient will look for and find occlusal discrepancies in that he can move the mandible in a thousand positions. The minute he starts showing signs or symptoms of a positive occlusal sense, you should make him a nightguard appliance to take his mind off his changed occlusion. A wise practitioner may refer this patient to another doctor.

ADDITIONAL CONSIDERATIONS

Pulpal pathosis can cause a tooth to be in trauma. Such a tooth may not be endodontically symptomatic. The pulpal involvement could be caused by trauma, a crack in the tooth, or a furcation involvement from a periodontal pocket. When an isolated tooth is in trauma and mobile, check the vitality of the tooth to rule out pulpal pathosis.

When worn-out defective restorations cannot be adjusted to establish centric holding stops, they should be replaced.

Occlusal adjustments will not stabilize teeth that have no opposing occlusal contacts. For example, lower second molars that do not have opposing maxillary second molars will overerupt and create occlusal disharmonies; if they are adjusted, the result will not be permanent.

Occlusal disharmonies associated with myofunctional habits such as tongue thrusting cannot be resolved until the habit is eliminated.

Occlusal adjustments will not correct occlusal disharmonies caused by improperly contoured crowns that impinge on the neutral zone of the teeth. For example, an anterior maxillary crown that extends 2 mm farther labially than the original tooth impinges on the neutral zone of the orbicularis oris. The lip pulls this tooth back into a more lingual position, creating occlusal trauma. This problem should be corrected by making a properly contoured crown rather than by continuing to grind out the lingual surface of this crown. Otherwise you will probably cut through the entire crown and into the tooth.

Restorative Dentistry

One of the major local irritants to gingival tissues is defective restorative dentistry. The most conservative restoration to accomplish the desired protection for a tooth and the periodontium is the restoration of choice. Restorations must fulfil three basic requirements if they are to complement the results of periodontal therapy: (1) They must be cleansable by the patient. They should have proper contours with

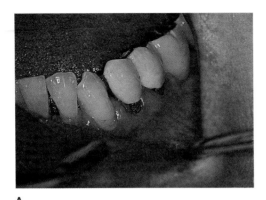
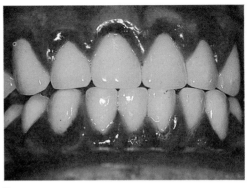

A   B

FIGURE 8–7 • Damage caused by restorations with subgingival margins. (A) Fixed bridge replacing first molar. Margins were originally subgingival, but plaque retention, inflammation, and subsequent destruction of the supporting tissues caused recession. Note buccal margins had to be restored with amalgam because of subgingival caries. (B) Periodontal damage in 18-year-old male caused by crowns with deep subgingival margins. The crowns were made because of tetracycline staining.

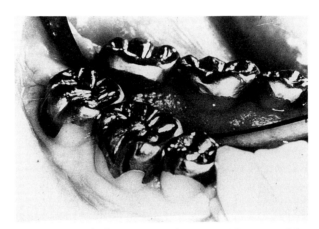

FIGURE 8–8 • Ideal restorative dentistry. Where possible, supragingival margins have been used to allow flossing. Good contacts and a stable coordinated occlusion has allowed this patient to function for 18 years without any wear faceting. Supragingival margins such as these are the kindest of all to the gingival tissue. Note that the mandibular second and first molars both have three buccal cusps. This develops an idling groove which allows the mesiobuccal cusps of the maxillary molars to move through without creating nonfunctional interference. (Courtesy Dr. Peter K. Thomas)

good accessible margins that are supragingival where possible. Subgingival margins will initially cause inflammation, which usually leads to bone loss (Fig. 8–7). (2) They must restore a stable, functional occlusion if the occlusal surfaces are involved. (Firm contact areas help ensure stability.) (3) They must protect the integrity of the cusps to prevent fractures (that is, they should be onlays instead of inlays). The restoration which usually best fulfills these three requirements for posterior teeth is the cast gold onlay with supragingivally placed margins (Fig. 8–8). Because of old existing restorations, full coverage is sometimes necessary on posterior teeth. To

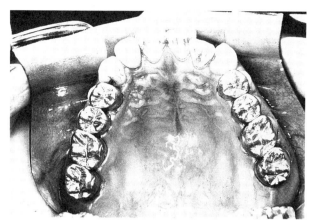

FIGURE **8–9** • Ideal restorative dentistry. Note that the occlusal table width of the molars is the same as that of the premolars. With multiple restorations contacts should be made tighter than required: the teeth will move when temporaries are in place, so that permanent restorations will have to reestablish bracing contacts.

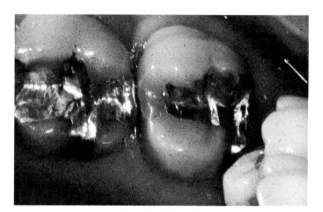

FIGURE **8–10** • Properly placed amalgam.

obtain flossable interproximal margins with cast gold onlays or crowns, we have found that a box preparation with a long bevel works best. Dr. Peter K. Thomas' technique of finishing buccal and lingual margins before and during cementation is excellent.

To restore open contacts of a posterior segment, temporarily cement one mesio-occlusal distal onlay or crown and recement it weekly after adding gold solder to the contact areas to orthodontically move the teeth closer together in the entire area (Fig. 8–9). The occlusion changes with this treatment and frequent occlusal adjustments are necessary. A quicker and simpler way to restore open contacts is to place a rubber separation medium in the center of the problematic area, then place permanent restorations after the teeth move.

Amalgams should have tight contacts, good occlusion, and good interproximal contours. They should be modified or replaced when they interfere with proper oral hygiene (Figs. 8–10, 8–11, 8–12).

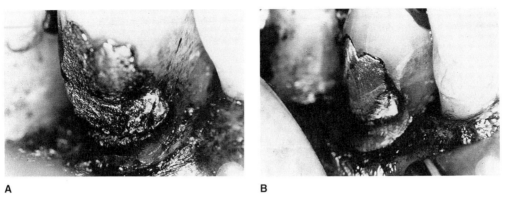

A

B

FIGURE **8–11** • Amalgams. (*A*) Subgingival amalgam margin after surgical exposure. (*B*) Appearance after root planing and smoothing of old amalgam to eliminate plaque retention.

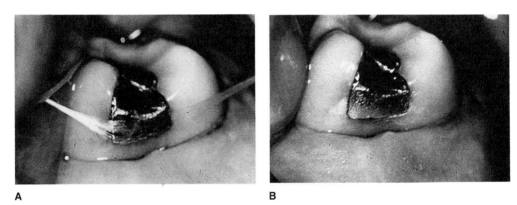

A

B

FIGURE **8–12** • Amalgams. (*A*) Floss shredding on an overhanging amalgam margin. (*B*) Same margin after smoothing with EVA diamond.

Fixed Bridges

All the requirements for gold onlays apply to fixed bridges. When properly made and maintained, fixed bridges are the most comfortable, serviceable, and lasting replacement available. However, if the margins are not right, the bridge is only as strong as the cement used to place it. We concur with Dr. Peter K. Thomas that it is impossible to cement more than three castings at one time and get each all the way into place when restoring teeth that were periodontically involved. Dr. Thomas uses key-way locks to unite large splints together and to avoid cementation of more than three abutments at a time (Fig. 8–13). A technique has been developed in Australia to obtain excellent porcelain margins for ceramo-metal crowns. In this technique a second die is used, the marginal area on the die is painted with cyanoacrylate, and then the porcelain receives a second firing to reline the margin. The resulting margins are as good as or better than cast gold onlay margins.

When a fixed bridge has been cemented, the patient should always be given floss threaders to allow the patient to floss the abutment teeth and under the pontics.

A fixed bridge is one of the most exacting restorations in dentistry and must be done properly. Otherwise the patient is better off with a partial denture.

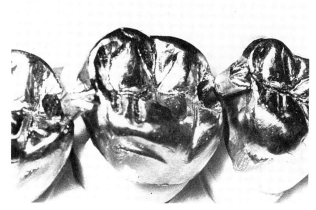

FIGURE **8–13** • Bridge made with keyway locks (Courtesy Dr. Peter K. Thomas).

Tooth-supported Denture

When only a few teeth remain and their prognosis is guarded, a tooth-supported denture should be considered. A poor crown-to-root ratio can be made favorable by endodontic therapy on the tooth followed by placement of a very short clinical crown. Connecting bars to splint the short copings aid in retaining the denture. It is important that the forces on the crowns be vertical and not horizontal. Therefore, when possible, only the occlusal surface should contact the denture.

Extractions

There are times when individual teeth should be extracted. The following are indications for extractions.

1. When a patient has a toothache and does not want to keep the tooth even though he is told it could be saved.
2. When a tooth has so little periodontal support that it cannot function painlessly and offers no help in the prognosis for the other teeth in its arch.
3. When a tooth prevents proper treatment of adjacent teeth and is not needed (malpositioned or root in close apposition to a key tooth needed for a fixed-bridge abutment).
4. When a tooth has a poor prognosis and the patient does not want to have much work or expense.
5. When all remaining teeth are doubtful. Many patients are best served in these circumstances by losing their maxillary teeth and having the lower teeth treated when possible. The prognosis for the lower teeth is improved greatly if the patient will sleep without the maxillary denture. However, most patients who are accustomed to sleeping with their maxillary denture cannot adjust to leaving it out and may need to wear a toothless night guard denture while sleeping (Fig. 8–14).
6. When a tooth has a deep osseous defect and would have a poor prognosis even if bone fill or bone graft were successful.

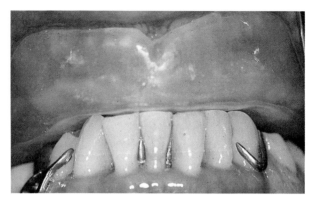

FIGURE 8–14 • Protection of edentulous maxillary tissue. This patient was asked to sleep without his maxillary full denture and mandibular partial denture. He began biting the edentulous maxillary tissue. Maxillary night guard was made for sleeping.

7. When a patient dislikes the appearance of a tooth so much that he wants it out and will not care about his other teeth until this one tooth is out (when a tooth is emotionally unacceptable).
8. When a tooth interferes with prosthetic needs (as in mandibular centrals and laterals when full lower splinting is indicated).
9. When the bone support of a tooth is being lost in such a manner that it is compromising the support of the adjacent tooth. This is especially an indication for extraction when the offending tooth is not critical to the overall prognosis for the dentition.

Partial Dentures

Partial dentures are often periodontal hazards but economic necessities. Given that many partials function for many years without causing periodontal pathosis, we

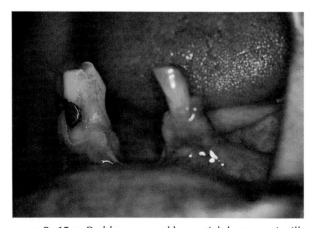

FIGURE 8–15 • Problems caused by partial dentures. An ill-fitting partial denture that had no occlusal or incisal rest was relined regularly because of settling. Note the tremendous destruction caused by this improperly designed replacement.

must study the characteristics of partial dentures that do cause problems so that we can avoid trouble (Fig. 8–15).

INDICATIONS FOR PARTIAL DENTURES

Partial dentures are indicated in the following circumstances:
1. When patients cannot afford fixed bridges.
2. When abutment teeth are likely to be lost in time.
3. When no posterior teeth are present.
4. When missing teeth are needed for masticating after fixed bridges have replaced all the teeth that are replaceable with fixed bridges.

OBJECTIVE FOR A PARTIAL DENTURE

To replace missing teeth.

CONSIDERATIONS FOR PARTIAL DENTURES

1. An accurate impression is essential.
2. Prepare occlusal rests only after surveying and designing the case.
3. For periodontally weak teeth that are mobile, prepare guide planes so that the teeth will be immobilized (Fig. 8–16).

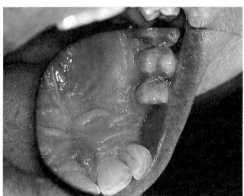

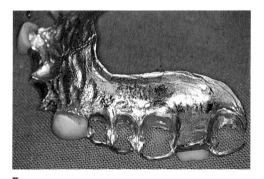

B

A

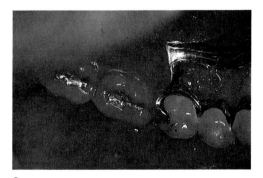

C

FIGURE **8–16** • Preparation for partial denture. (*A*) Teeth prepared for guide plane partial denture. Enamel is reshaped on the lingual to eliminate undercuts and to establish guide planes. (*B*) Multiple occlusal rests are added. (*C*) Guide plane partial denture inserted. If individual teeth are later lost, they can be repaired onto this partial denture. In 10 years no further loss of teeth has occurred.

4. Consider the prognosis of individual teeth when designing the partial so that future modifications can be made if and when individual teeth are lost.

5. On free-end saddle lower partials ensure complete coverage of the retromolar pads (Fig. 8–17).

6. Check that all saddles cover the masticatory functional gingival tissues but do not extend out onto the mucosa.

7. Ensure that the framework for free-end saddles has a metal posterior contact with the model to prevent dislodgement of framework on the model when acrylic is packed, flasked, and processed.

8. Ensure that occlusal rests and replaced teeth do not occlude harder than patient's teeth unless opening of the bite is indicated.

9. Test occlusal contacts of replaced teeth with shimstock.

10. Ideally, have a cast gold occlusion on replaced teeth contacting natural

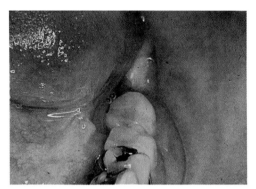
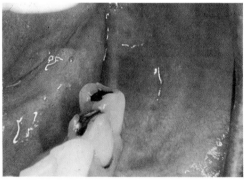

A   B

FIGURE 8–17 • Design of partial dentures. (A) This mandibular partial denture does not properly cover the retromolar pads and extends out into mucosal tissues. (B) Inflammation caused by the denture.

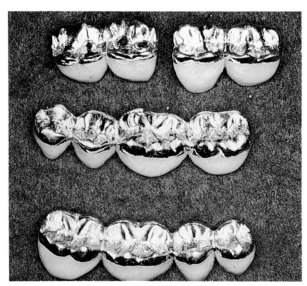

FIGURE 8–18 • Cast gold occlusal pontics to be used on a partial denture. (Courtesy Dr. J. Meeks)

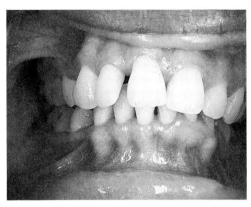 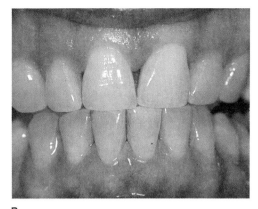

A   B

FIGURE **8–19** • Minor tooth movement. (*A*) Appearance after gingivectomy on the right side of the maxilla. (*B*) Appearance after both sides had been operated.

teeth (Fig. 8–18). If the patient cannot afford this, use acrylic teeth and place occlusal amalgams to prevent excessive wear.

11. When designing a partial denture for an arch containing weakened teeth that are essential to the stability of the prosthesis, make the path of insertion parallel to the long axis of the weakened key tooth to prevent lateral forces during insertion, removal, and function of the appliance.

12. Instruct patients always to insert partials with their hands and never to bite them into place. The reason is that in designing a case it is usually necessary to tip the model in some direction to create undercuts for retention. Therefore, a partial should not be forced into place by biting it because doing so will either loosen the clasped teeth or loosen the clasps. This is why so many patients keep coming back for adjustments to loose clasps.

13. Give the patient a clasp brush.

Minor Tooth Movement

Teeth that have moved out of position because of loss of periodontal supporting tissues sometimes realign themselves after periodontal therapy. Many times, however, they stay in their abnormal position (Fig. 8–19). If the teeth were straight before the periodontal breakdown, it is helpful to realign them back into contact with their adjacent teeth to improve appearance and help develop bracing contacts (Fig. 8–20). It may be necessary to stabilize the teeth in their proper position by bonding them with composite restorative material or by using a night-guard appliance to act as a retainer. The many techniques for tooth movement are adequately described in textbooks.

INDICATIONS FOR MINOR TOOTH MOVEMENT

Minor tooth movement is indicated in the following circumstances:
    1. When patients are concerned about their appearance.

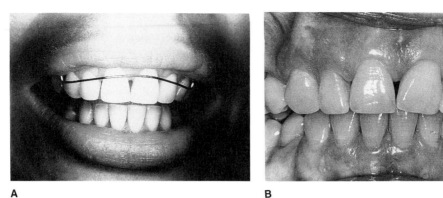

A   **B**

FIGURE **8–20** • Minor tooth movement, same patient as Fig. 8-19. (A) Modified Hawley bite plane in place for minor tooth movement. (B) Appearance 30 years later. Note papillary regeneration when compared with immediate postoperative view.

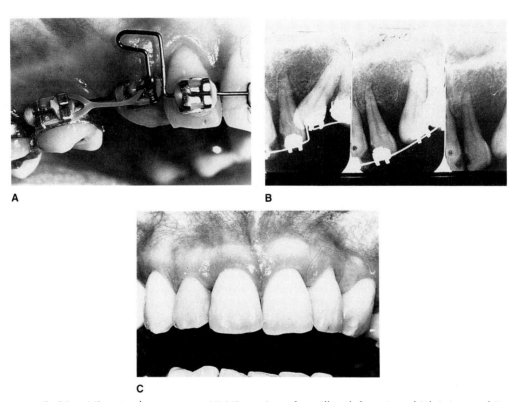

A   **B**

C

FIGURE **8–21** • Minor tooth movement. (A) Mirror view of maxillary left canine which is in crossbite and linguoversion and has a 7 mm pocket on the mesial aspect. (B) Radiographic appearance of canine immediately after bonding, 8 months later, and 1 year later (the orthodontic appliance was removed). (C) Postoperative appearance. Left canine is out of crossbite. Tooth movement resolved the pocket on the mesial aspect by correcting the cementoenamel junction discrepancy with the lateral.

2. When teeth are not stable due to lack of bracing contacts.
3. When tooth malposition is causing a periodontal pocket (Fig. 8–21).
4. When a tooth must be placed in parallel to be used in a fixed bridge or fixed splint (Fig. 8–22).
5. When open contacts that cause food impaction must be closed.

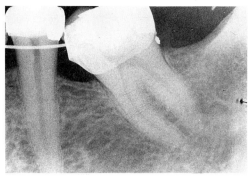 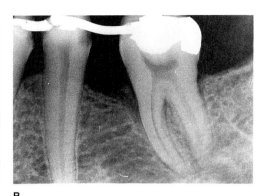

A   B

FIGURE **8–22** • Minor tooth movement. (A) Radiograph of molar banded for uprighting. (B) Molar uprighted in preparation for a fixed bridge. (Courtesy Drs. Manuel H. Marks and Herman Corn)

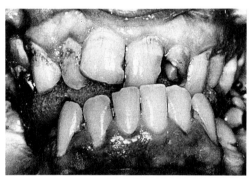 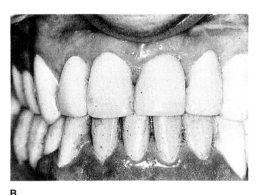

A   B

FIGURE **8–23** • Minor tooth movement. (A) Decayed, malposed teeth with poor gingival contours and inflammation. Patient received periodontal and orthodontic therapy, as well as prosthetic therapy consisting of temporary restorations. (B) Postoperative appearance with temporary crowns. (Courtesy Dr. Edwin S. Rosenberg)

OBJECTIVES FOR MINOR TOOTH MOVEMENT

1. To improve appearance (Fig. 8–23).
2. To restore bracing contacts to stabilize teeth.
3. To help use a tooth for a fixed bridge or splint rather than extract the tooth (Fig. 8–24).
4. To restore tooth-to-tooth contact bracing to prevent food impaction.

Fixed Splinting

Fixed splinting entails the uniting of crowns or onlays so that teeth weakened from secondary occlusal trauma can be stabilized to prevent mobility. Unfortunately, splinting creates problems for the patient's oral hygiene and may interfere with the normal physiologic mesial drift of the teeth.

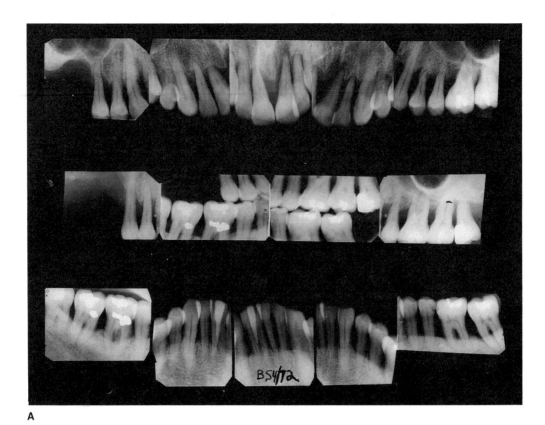

A

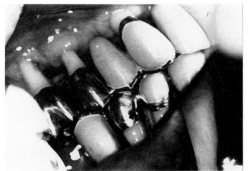

B

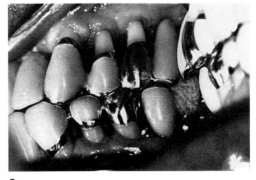

C

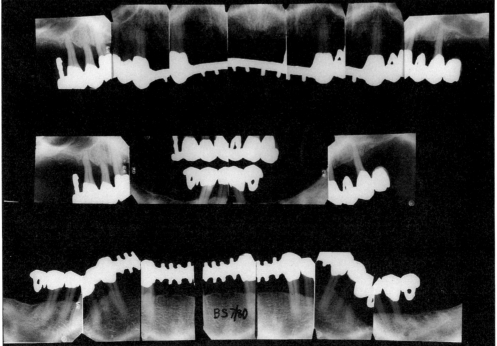

142 **D**

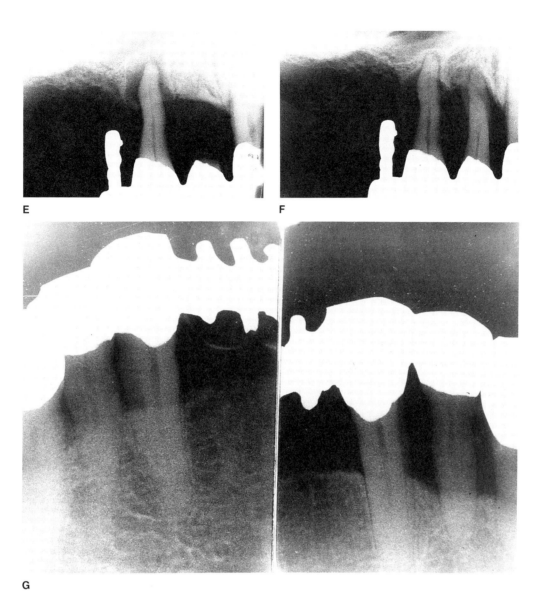

E

F

G

FIGURE 8–24 • Fixed splinting. (*A*) Advanced generalized periodontitis. Patient had secondary occlusal trauma with Class 2 or 3 mobility on all teeth. (*B*) After periodontal surgery temporary fixed splints were constructed (courtesy Dr. G. Ronald Bradley). (*C*) Same patient other side. Patient was told that prognosis was poor and that 5–6 years' use was all that could be expected. (*D*) Appearance 8 years after surgery. (*E*) Upper right area 10 years after surgery, before sacrifice of the first premolar. (*F*) Same area 2 years later (12 years after surgery). Second premolar was sacrificed. Patient then went to a maxillary partial denture, which lasted 2 years before he went to a full upper denture (14 years after the original surgery). (*G*) Mandibular teeth 14 years after surgery.

INDICATIONS FOR FIXED SPLINTING

1. Secondary occlusal trauma for all the remaining teeth in an arch. Secondary occlusal trauma is trauma caused by normal occlusal forces to the attachment apparatus of teeth weakened by the loss of supporting mechanisms.
2. When so many teeth are to be replaced with fixed bridges that splinting cannot be avoided (e.g., when only the canines and second molars are present).

3. When a partial denture is to be avoided and additional teeth are needed for mastication. An example would be the splinting of canine, first premolar, and second premolar to cantilever a small pontic shaped like a third premolar.

OBJECTIVES OF FIXED SPLINTING

1. To establish cross-arch stabilization so that primary forces are in a vertical rather than a lateral direction.
2. To replace missing teeth with fixed bridges rather than a partial denture when only a few teeth remain.
3. To provide the comfort of a fixed bridge rather than a partial denture.

CONSIDERATIONS IN FIXED SPLINTING

1. Make crowns so that they are cleanable (open embrasures, exposed supragingival margins when possible).
2. When possible, design the fixed splinting so that if individual teeth are later lost the fixed splint can be modified with only minor procedures. Permanent cementation of copings on each tooth and temporary cementation of the fixed splint allows easy removal of the splint for modifications. Key-way interlocks can be used to prepare for future modifications caused by loss of an individual tooth in a long splint
3. Always use all caries-prevention procedures to avoid caries around the crowns.

CONTRAINDICATIONS FOR FIXED SPLINTS

1. A patient who cannot or will not achieve a very high degree of plaque control.
2. A patient who cannot afford the costs entailed by the many hours and expenses of this type of therapy.
3. A patient who is not willing to make the extreme efforts necessary to accomplish fixed splinting. Patients must be informed about all the complications involved and the need for close supervised maintenance follow-up care.

Night-guard Appliances

Most young people grind their teeth in their sleep to some degree when teeth are erupting. A few continue to brux and cause excessive wearing of the occlusal and incisal surfaces. Bruxism also loosens teeth and causes primary occlusal trauma. If occlusal adjustments to eliminate centric prematurities and nonfunctional interferences do not stop bruxism, autosuggestion should be tried. With autosuggestion, a patient tells himself at night before going to bed that if he grinds or clenches his

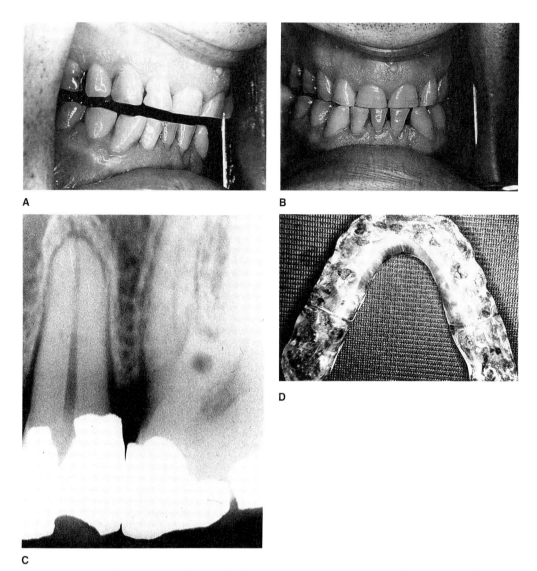

FIGURE 8–25 • Night guard appliances for bruxism. (A) Severe attrition of teeth due to bruxism. (B) Same patient. Note lack of incisal guidance. (C) Same patient. Note root resorption and increased sclerosis of the bone due to heavy occlusal forces. (D) Night guard for same patient. It is flat and balanced in all directions, like the patient's occlusion.

teeth, he will awaken and relax his teeth apart and go back to sleep. If he does awaken, he must restate his autosuggestion for it to work again. Some patients awaken ten to fifteen times the first night and not at all or only once or twice after that. Autosuggestion works best for people who awaken each morning before hearing the alarm clock.

If autosuggestion is not effective, an appliance should be made to mitigate the damage of bruxism by directing all forces on the teeth in a vertical direction rather than horizontally. If less than 3 mm of anterior vertical overlap of the incisal edges is present in centric occlusion, a maxillary or mandibular flat plane appliance should be used (Fig. 8–25). If more than 3 mm of overlap is present, a modified Hawley bite plane made to be within free way space should be used if the anterior teeth are not mobile. If the anterior teeth are mobile, a Hawley bite plane is made with an

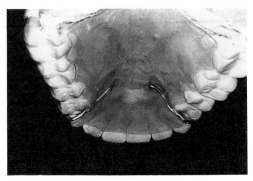
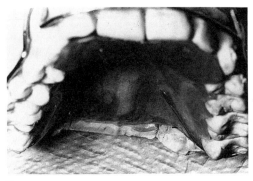

A   **B**

FIGURE 8–26 • Night guard appliances for bruxism. (*A*) Maxillary Hawley bite plane night guard. This guard must be adjusted to occlude with the mandibular anterior teeth and be as perpendicular as possible to the long axis of the mandibular anterior teeth. The posterior teeth should not occlude in centric or any excursions and should be within the freeway space limitations. A problem that may develop with this appliance is that the labial arch wire can settle between the first premolar and canine, causing the contact between these teeth to open. (*B*) To avoid opening contacts by crossing the occlusion, a heavy arch wire and a wire from the distal side of the arch that do not cross the occlusion are used.

anterior platform to occlude within the free way space and an occluding flat plane to cover the posterior teeth (Fig. 8–26).

Vitamin and Mineral Supplements

If a patient receiving periodontal therapy does not have a well-balanced diet containing adequate protein, vitamins, and minerals, he will not obtain the best results possible. Good nutrition also helps to prevent future problems. The addition of a good combination vitamin and mineral supplement may be all that is required. If, however, a patient has symptoms of medical complications, he must see his physician. Do not prescribe calcium for your patients, but have them consult their physician on dosage, and so on. The reason is that some patients can develop kidney stones if they take calcium. Suggest multiple vitamins not to exceed the suggested daily minimum requirements.

Postoperative Sequelae

Many postoperative problems can occur after corrective periodontal therapy. The most common are pain, bleeding, swelling, and infection. Proper patient selection and sound surgical techniques will prevent most of these problems.

Pain can usually be well controlled by giving the patient ibuprofen 600 mg starting in the morning and continuing every 4 hours on the day of surgery (not to exceed 3200 mg per day total dose). Careful, gentle handling of the tissues will help minimize postoperative pain and trauma.

When even small areas of bone are exposed postoperatively some patients will get symptoms resembling those caused by dry socket and localized alveolar osteitis.

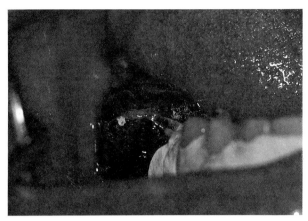

FIGURE **8–27** • Postoperative sequelae. Abnormal (liver) clot 8 hours after surgery. Clot was removed, area was cauterized, and vitamin K was injected intramuscularly.

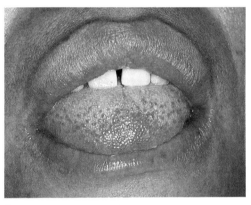
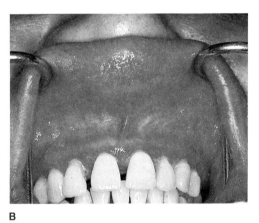

A   **B**

FIGURE **8–28** • Postoperative sequelae. (*A*) Swollen tongue and lips from an allergy to eugenol in periodontal dressing. (*B*) Erythema in same patient from allergy. Dressing was changed to non-eugenol type and 50 mg diphenhydramine b.i.d. was used to resolve the problem.

In our experience, iodoform gauze wetted with eugenol, placed on the area and held over it with periodontal pack will greatly alleviate the patient's discomfort.

When postoperative bleeding occurs, treat initially with pressure. Abnormal clots may need to be removed to stop bleeding (Fig. 8–27). Vitamin K injected intramuscularly is often helpful in controlling postoperative bleeding.

Allergies to medications and dressings may cause postoperative problems, in which case the offending agent should be removed and antihistamines or steroids should be prescribed (Fig. 8–28).

Internal or external root resorption can occur during the maintenance phase of periodontal therapy. This is another justification for periodic radiography in the maintenance of patients (Fig. 8–29).

Postoperative root sensitivity is a perplexing problem to both patient and doctor. Dry burnishing is a most helpful treatment. The technique is described in Chapter 9 (see Fig. 9–7).

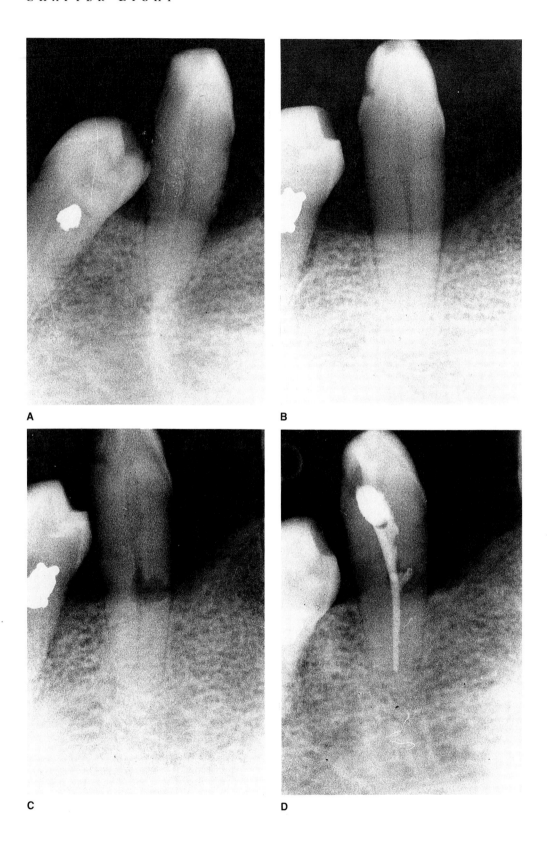

A

B

C

D

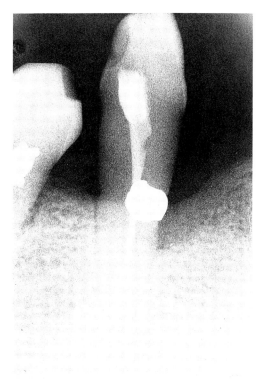

E

FIGURE 8–29 • Postoperative sequelae. (A) Preoperative radiograph of mandibular canine. Bony defect is evident on mesial surface. (B) Appearance 1 month after surgery. Freeze-dried demineralized bone was placed into the defect. (C) Appearance 5 years after surgery. The graft has become more radiopaque as it healed and matured. However, there is radiographic evidence of internal resorption. (D) Root canal therapy was performed. (E) Area was treated with apically positioned flap and removal of 2 mm of bone so restoration could be placed in the area of resorption. (Courtesy Drs. David Morris and Dewey Newbold)

Bibliography

Alfano MC. Controversies, perspectives, and clinical implications of nutrition in periodontal disease. Dent Clin North Am 1976; 20:519–548.

Bergenholtz G, Nyman S. Endodontic complications following periodontal and prosthetic treatment of patients with advanced periodontal disease. J Periodontol 1984; 55:63–68.

Chin Quee TA, et al. Surgical removal of the fully impacted mandibular third molar: The influence of flap design and alveolar bone height on the periodontal status of the second molar. J Periodontol 1985; 56:625–630.

Courtade GL, Timmermans JJ. Pins in restorative dentistry. St. Louis: CV Mosby, 1971.

Curtis JW, et al. The incidence and severity of complications and pain following periodontal surgery. J Periodontol 1985; 56:597–601.

Ericsson I, Lindhe J. Lack of significance of increased tooth mobility in experimental periodontits. J Periodontol 1984; 55:447–452.

Kaufman H, et al. The influence of trauma from occlusion on the bacterial repopulation of periodontal pockets in dogs. J Periodontol 1984; 55:86–92.

Kerry GJ, et al. Effect of periodontal treatment on tooth mobility. J Periodontol 1982; 53:635–638.

Lamster IB, et al. Rapid loss of alveolar bone associated with nonprecious alloy crowns in two patients with nickel hypersensitivity. J Periodontol 1987; 58:486–492.

Larato DC. The effect of crown margin extension on gingival inflammation. J South Calif State Dent Assoc 1969; 37:476–478.

Lindhe J, Svanberg G. Influence of trauma from occlusion on progression of experimental periodontitis in the beagle dog. J Clin Periodontol 1974; 1:3–14.

Manor A, et al. "Spontaneous" repositioning of migrated teeth following periodontal surgery. J Clin Periodontol 1984; 11:540–545.

Marino VA, et al. Severe localized destruction of the periodontium secondary to subgingival displacement of an elastic band. Report of a case. J Periodontol 1988; 57:472–477.

Marks MH, Corn H. Atlas of adult orthodontics. Philadelphia: Lea & Febiger, 1988.

Morrow R, Handbook of immediate overdentures. St. Louis, C. V. Mosby, 1978.

Nyman S, Ericsson I. The capacity of reduced periodontal tissue to support fixed bridgework. J Clin Periodontol 1982; 9:409–414.

O'Leary TJ, Standish SM, Bloomer RS. Severe periodontal destruction following impression procedures. J Periodontol 1973; 44:43–48.

Pihlstrom BL, et al. Association between signs of trauma from occlusion and periodontitis. J Periodontol 1986; 57:1–6.

Polson AM, Meitner SW, Zander HA. Trauma and progression of marginal periodontitis in squirrel monkeys. IV. Reversibility of bone loss due to trauma alone and trauma superimposed upon periodontitis. J Periodont Res 1976; 11:290–298.

Polson AM, Reed BE. Long-term effect of orthodontic treatment on crestal alveolar bone levels. J Periodontol 1984; 55:28–34.

Ramfjord SP, Ash MM. Occlusion. 2nd ed. Philadelphia: WB Saunders, 1971.

Ramfjord SP, Ash MM Jr. Significance of occlusion in the etiology and treatment of early, moderate and advanced periodontitis. J Periodontol 1981; 52:511–517.

Roulet JF, Roulet-Mehrens TK. The surface roughness of restorative materials and dental tissues after polishing with prophylaxis and polishing pastes. J Periodontol 1982; 53:257–266.

Sheffler GJ, McFall WT Jr. Occlusal relations and periodontal status in human adults. J Periodontol 1984; 55:368–374.

Silness J. Periodontal conditions in patients treated with dental bridges. III. The relationship between the location of the crown margins and the periodontal condition. J Periodont Res 1970; 5:225–229.

Stetler KJ, Bissada NF. Significance of the width of keratinized gingiva on the periodontal status of teeth with submarginal restorations. J Periodontol 1987; 58:696–700.

Stuart CE. Occlusal adjustments. In: Huffman RW, Gegenos JW, eds. Principles of occlusion. London, Ohio: H & R Press, 1973.

Than A, et al. Relationship between restorations and the level of the periodontal attachment. J Clin Periodontol 1982; 9:193–202.

Thomas PK, Syllabus on Full Mouth Waxing, Technique for Rehabilitation, Tooth-to-Tooth, Clasp Fossa Concept of Organic Occlusion, 2nd ed. School of Dentistry, Postgraduate Education, University of California, Los Angeles, 1967.

Vogel RI, Gross JI. The effects of nonsteroidal anti-inflammatory analgesics on pain after periodontal surgery. J Am Dent Assoc 1984; 109:731–734.

Williams WN, et al. The effect of periodontal bone loss on bite force discrimination. J Periodontol 1987; 58:236–239.

Yuodelis RA, Weaver JD, Sapkos S. Facial and lingual contours of artificial complete crown restorations and their effects on the periodontium. J Prosthet Dent 1973; 29:61–66.

CHAPTER NINE

Patient Instruction, Maintenance of the Treated Case, and Long-Term Results

Patients who have undergone periodontal therapy should return for follow-up treatments every 3 to 6 months. In our experience a longer interval than that can lead to serious problems, because patients tend to stop flossing completely and lose interest in their oral hygiene.

A survey of 100 consecutive patients in our practice yielded the following results: Fifty-eight of those surveyed flossed twice a day. These patients were easily maintained for the most part. Thirty patients flossed an average of once a day. A few of these were difficult to maintain, but most were maintaining well. Twelve patients flossed only once or twice a week. Of these, six maintained well and the other six constantly developed problems such as abscesses and so on. These statistics emphasize what we all know: the long-range success of periodontal therapy depends on the patient becoming proficient in his oral hygiene procedures.

Oral Hygiene Instructions for Patients

It cannot be overemphasized to the patient that the long-term success of periodontal therapy depends on how well the patient performs his oral hygiene procedures. Since no one method is effective for all patients, the clinician must determine which techniques are best for the individual and instruct him carefully. Periodontal therapy and other dental treatment can then have long-lasting results.

Several appointments for chair-side instructions are needed before the average patient can visualize the prescribed method so that he can actually follow it. One period of instruction in dental flossing and toothbrushing, given by skilled personnel, results in only 50% retention and application by highly intelligent persons. This is an optimum result; the average result is nearer 25%. Patients frequently state that they "forgot" part of the instructions or "thought" they were carrying out the procedures in the manner that the clinician demonstrated.

Most patients are deficient in interproximal cleaning of teeth. A number of methods and devices commonly used for this purpose can be evaluated. In our experience unwaxed dental floss yields the best results.

Two acceptable methods of toothbrushing are the modified roll and the Bass techniques. Either one of these methods, or a combination of the two, is effective for most clinical situations; and most patients achieve a high degree of proficiency. Other methods are also effective. If you find on initial examination that the patient is achieving an acceptable result with the method he is using with no evidence of hard or soft tissue damage, do not attempt to change it.

The modified roll technique is especially indicated for labial and buccal surfaces, if tissue contours are fairly normal, and if recessions or erosions are present. If the patient is accustomed to overvigorous horizontal brushing, he is more likely to change to the modified roll technique than the Bass technique. We start all new patients on the modified roll technique, but change to the Bass technique after pocket elimination if the patient is unable to maintain clean teeth. The Bass technique is especially effective for the lingual surfaces of mandibular teeth; in the presence of tori, exostosis, or irregular contours; and when Class V caries is prevalent. If, after a reasonable period, the patient is not achieving an acceptable result with one technique, the other should be used, in whole or in part.

Instruct patients in effective oral hygiene by warning them about bacterial plaque in the following terms:

> One of the major causes of tooth decay and periodontal (gum) disease is bacterial plaque. Bacterial plaque is an almost invisible film of decomposed food particles and millions of living bacteria in a sticky material that is not water soluble. To prevent dental disease this destructive film must be removed every day. Keeping your teeth clean and healthy will promote better general health and help you preserve your natural appearance, enjoy chewing and talking, and prevent bad breath.

USE OF DENTAL FLOSS

For most people dental decay and periodontal diseases occur primarily *between* the teeth. The toothbrush cannot effectively clean these areas or behind the last tooth in each arch. Unwaxed dental floss is most effective for cleaning these areas, and patients with bone loss should use it at least twice a day—after breakfast and after the last meal of the day. Once a day is sufficient for patients who do not have bone loss.

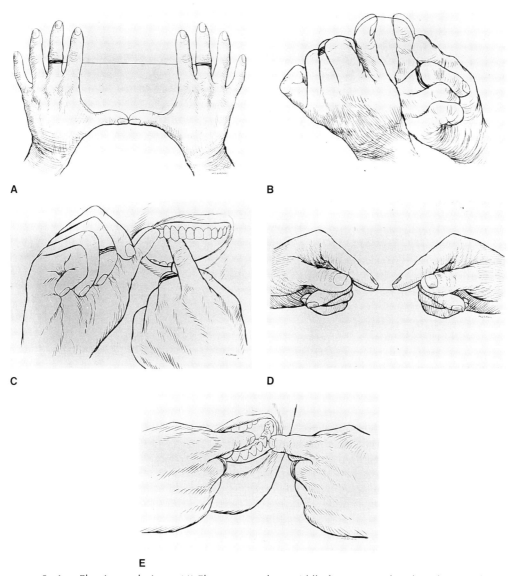

A

B

C

D

E

FIGURE **9–1** • Flossing technique. (*A*) Floss wrapped on middle fingers. (*B*) Thumb to the outside for upper teeth. (*C*) Flossing between upper back teeth. (*D*) Holding floss for lower teeth. (*E*) Flossing between lower back teeth.

Suggestions for Flossing

1. Cut off a piece of floss about 3 feet long. Lightly wrap the ends of the floss around the middle joint of your middle fingers as shown in Figure 9–1 A.
2. Keep the fingers controlling the floss not more than one-half inch apart.
3. Do not force the floss between the teeth. Insert it gently by sawing back and forth at the point where the teeth contact each other. Let it slide gently into place.

4. With *both* fingers move the floss up and down with moderate pressure six times on the side of one tooth, and then repeat on the side of the other tooth until the surfaces are "squeaky" clean.

5. Go to the gum tissue with the floss, but not into the gum so as to cause discomfort, soreness, or bleeding.

6. When the floss becomes frayed or soiled, turn from one middle finger to the other to bring up a fresh section.

7. To clean between the *upper left back* teeth pass the floss over your *left* thumb and *right* forefinger (Fig. 9–1 B).

8. To clean between the *upper right* teeth pass the floss over your *right* thumb and *left* forefinger. To see the proper position of the hands, look at Figure 9–1 C. The thumb is to the outside of the teeth, and helps hold the cheek back. Now the *right* thumb is outside the teeth and the *left* forefinger is on the inside.

9. To clean between all *lower* teeth hold the floss with the forefingers of both hands (Fig. 9–1 D). You will be able to insert the floss gently between all *lower* teeth with the floss over your forefingers in this position. Figure 9–1 E shows the correct method for flossing between the *lower* back teeth, using the two forefingers to guide the floss.

At first, flossing may be awkward and slow, but continued practice will increase skill and effectiveness.

Rinsing

Rinse vigorously with water after flossing to remove food particles and plaque that you have cut loose. When you are unable to floss or brush after eating, rinse with water. Rinsing alone will not remove the organized bacterial plaque but helps to remove food particles. Also, water-irrigating devices alone will not remove the organized bacterial plaque because it is not water soluble (Fig. 9–2).

TOOTHBRUSHING

The toothbrush will remove the bacterial film from the outer, the inner, and the biting surfaces of the teeth. Brush gently, but with enough pressure to feel the bristles on the gum. Do not use so much pressure that you feel discomfort. The following method is effective and relatively easy for most patients. Sometimes another method is recommended in special situations, such as crooked teeth.

Toothpaste foams and prevents you from seeing if the brush is placed properly. While learning to brush properly it is best to omit the use of toothpaste or to use it in a second brushing.

Modified Roll Technique

Most patients are started on the modified roll technique of brushing as it is a complete change from scrubbing the teeth. Also, it helps keep pocket exudates expressed into the mouth, thereby preventing a blockage of the orifice of the pocket that could cause an acute periodontal abscess.

For the *outer* surface of all teeth, place the brush on the gum tissue at a 45-degree angle. Then sweep slowly over the gum tissue and teeth. (Look care-

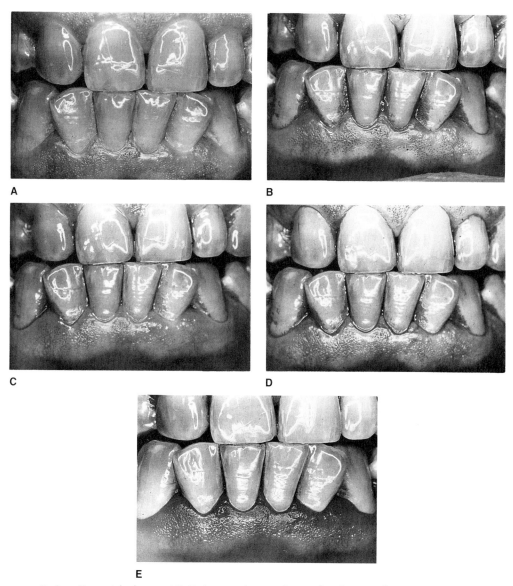

FIGURE 9–2 • Bacterial plaque. (*A*) Patient 72 hours after no brushing or flossing. (*B*) Appearance after staining. Note plaque. (*C*) Same patient after using water irrigator. (*D*) Appearance after staining. Plaque is still present. (*E*) Teeth stained after flossing and brushing.

fully at Figure 9–3.) On the *upper* teeth, sweep downward only. On the *lower* teeth, sweep upward only. Brushing slowly lets the tips of the bristles thoroughly remove the film from the junction between the gum tissue and the tooth.

Use the same technique for the *inside* surface of the *upper back* teeth (Fig. 9–4 A). For the *inside* surface of the *lower back* teeth, set the brush where the teeth join the gums and make several back-and-forth strokes over the teeth and gums (study Fig. 9–4 B). For the *inside* surface of the *upper front* teeth, hold the brush vertically as in Figure 9–4 C and sweep downward over the gum tissue and teeth. For the *lower front* teeth, sweep upward over the gum tissue and teeth (Figure 9–4 D).

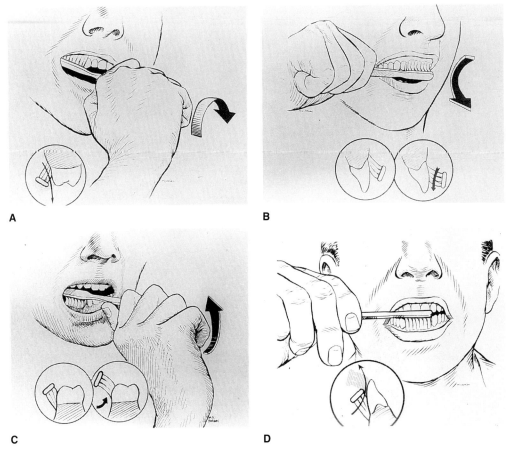

FIGURE 9–3 • Brushing outer surfaces, modified roll technique. (*A*) Hold brush at 45-degree angle. (*B*) On upper teeth, sweep downward. (*C*) On lower teeth, sweep upward. (*D*) Always sweep from the gums over the teeth.

The brush can effectively reach only one or two teeth at one placement. Change the position of the brush as often as is necessary to adequately reach and clean all tooth surfaces. Six strokes at each brush placement are usually sufficient. To clean the *biting* surfaces, brush back and forth as shown in Figure 9–5.

After brushing, rinse vigorously to remove the loosened plaque from the teeth and mouth.

Bass Technique

When the modified roll technique is not indicated or does not achieve the desired results, substitute the Bass technique in whole or in part. When deep periodontal pockets have been eliminated by resective surgical procedures, less than ideal contours often result. The Bass brushing technique is then usually indicated. Many patients learn to combine the Bass technique with the modified roll technique.

For the *outside* surface of all teeth and the *inside* surface of the back teeth, position the brush with the bristles at the junction between the teeth and gums (study Fig. 9–6 A); note the exact position of the brush. Then move the brush back and forth with short strokes several times as in Figure 9-6 B–G. Study each figure carefully.

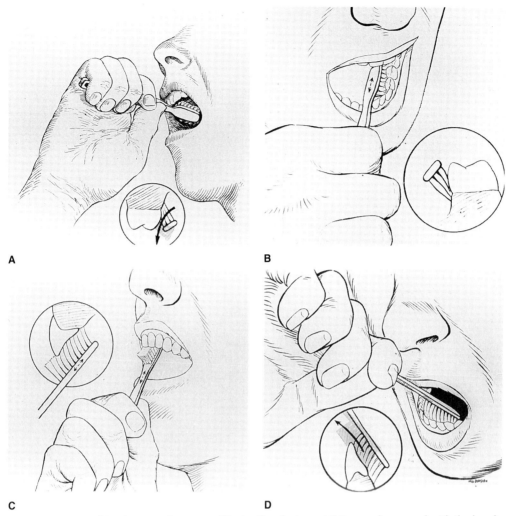

A   B

C   D

FIGURE 9–4 • Brushing inner surfaces, modified roll technique. (*A*) Sweep downward with the brush. (*B*) Brush carefully *back* and *forth*. (*C*) Sweep *downward* over upper gums and teeth. (*D*) Sweep *upward* over lower gums and teeth.

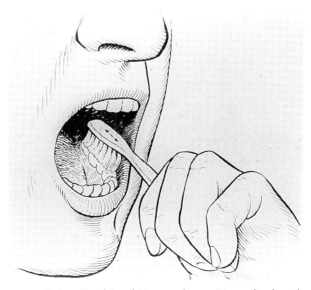

FIGURE 9–5 • Brushing biting surfaces. Use a back-and-forth motion.

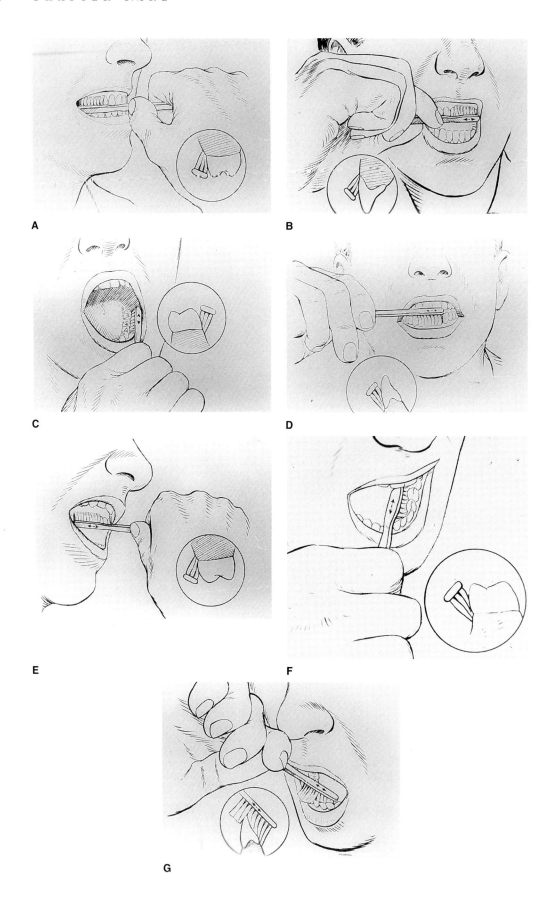

A

B

C

D

E

F

G

FIGURE **9–6** • The Bass technique for toothbrushing. (*A*) Place brush where teeth and gums meet. (*B*) Move the brush as shown by arrows. (*C*) Keep brush where teeth and gums meet. (*D*) Use short careful strokes. (*E*) Use same method on inside surfaces. (*F*) Brush back and forth. (*G*) Keep strokes short.

For the *inside* surfaces of the *upper* and *lower front* teeth, hold the brush vertically as in Figure 9–6 G, and make several gentle back-and-forth strokes over the gum tissue and teeth.

To clean the *biting* surfaces, brush back and forth as in Figure 9–5.

The brush can effectively reach only one or two teeth at one placement. Change the position of the brush as often as is necessary to adequately reach and clean all tooth surfaces. After brushing, rinse vigorously to remove the loosened plaque from the teeth and mouth.

Some patients tend to overbrush or change from Bass brushing technique into scrubbing. Show them how to use only their thumb and forefinger in holding the brush.

Testing Teeth for Plaque

Give patients having difficulty in effectively controlling plaque a disclosing tablet. Have them chew the tablet until it is dissolved in their mouth, swish it vigorously around the teeth, and then empty their mouth. After they rinse with water, inspect their teeth. Red stains indicate areas where teeth are not completely clean. Explain to the patient that the red stain is held on the teeth by the bacterial plaque that the patient failed to remove in cleaning. For the patient's self-examination a small plastic dental mirror may be necessary.

Sensitive Teeth

After corrective periodontal treatments, exposed root surfaces are often sensitive to cold and heat. This condition usually only lasts for a few weeks or months if the teeth are kept meticulously clean. If the teeth are not kept clean, sensitivity will remain and become more severe. For the few patients who have severe sensitivity, continued special treatment will be needed.

The most effective method of treating root sensitivity is to first determine the precise area on the tooth which is causing the sensitivity. This is usually done using the tip of an explorer. An ice rod made in a discarded anesthetic carpule can be used if the explorer does not work. Once the area or areas are located, isolate the tooth with cotton rolls and gently dry it with a stream of air. Next burnish the area with a dry toothpick in a holder (Fig. 9–7). Then give the patient cool water to drink and ask him if he notices the difference. The procedure may need to be repeated, or other areas may be found. This treatment also works very well for patients who have self-induced root sensitivity from overzealous brushing.

This simple treatment is the most effective treatment for sensitivity that we have found in 50 years of combined practice. Patients with postsurgical root sensitivity are often disgruntled, and immediate resolution of their problem will change their entire attitude. Recall patients or new patients often present with root sensitivity problems and are impressed when you can solve a problem that others have not been able to manage. Your hygienist can be taught this simple technique, and it will be a great practice builder for you.

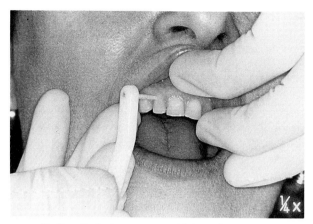

FIGURE 9–7 • Reducing root sensitivity. The sensitive area is being burnished with a dry toothpick in a holder. The tooth should also be dry.

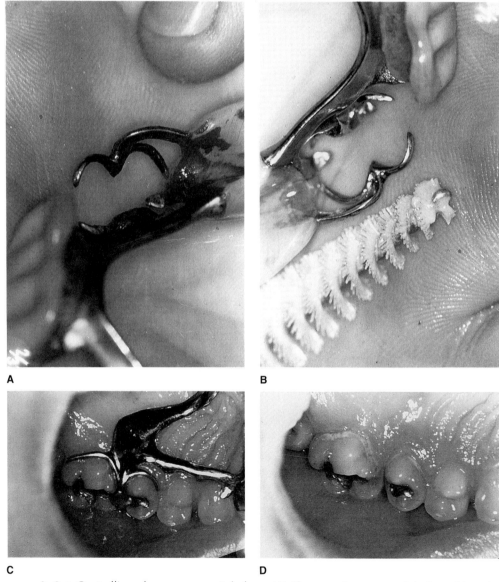

A

B

C

D

FIGURE 9–8 • Controlling plaque on a partial clasp. (A) Plaque stain on a partial clasp. Note the retained plaque on the inside of the clasp. (B) Butler clasp brush after cleaning partial. (C) Partial in place. (D) Decalcification on the enamel caused by clasp's plaque retention.

Special Aids for Special Problems

Oral hygiene can be maintained even when there are special difficulties. Partial clasps pose a particular problem in cleaning, and a clasp brush is required (Fig. 9–8). Cleaning plaque from the tongue also aids overall oral hygiene, and tongue scrapers are available. Allergic reactions to dentifrices can occasionally cause epithelial sloughing (Fig. 9–9). Such cases generally resolve when the dentifrice is changed to a bland type—typically the patient will have encountered the problem after changing brands of dentifrice, and the simplest remedy is to return to using the earlier brand. The patient should rinse with salt water until the condition resolves.

There are several toothpastes on the market which retard calculus formation. These dentifrices have pyrophosphate incorporated into them as the active ingredient. The commercial flavoring agent cinnamon aldehyde is used to cover up the salty taste of pyrophosphate, and its concentration has been increased dramatically over the concentration used in non-tartar control dentifrices. This has caused an

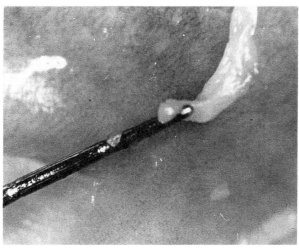

FIGURE **9–9** • Epithelial sloughing. This condition is usually caused by an allergic reaction to dentifrice.

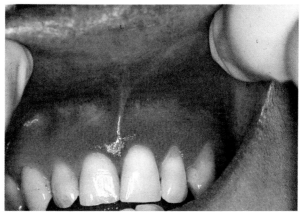

FIGURE **9–10** • Two face hypersensitivity reaction. Inflammation of facial gingiva and labial mucosa in a 32 year old female. (Courtesy Dr. Terry Rees)

allergic type gingivitis in a significant number of patients (Fig. 9–10). When the patient discontinues the use of the tartar control dentifrice the problem will usually correct itself within a matter of days (Fig. 9–11).

Special difficult-to-clean areas can often be reached by using a periodontal aid toothpick holder or special brush (Fig. 9–12). These devices can clean proximal concavities such as are seen on the maxillary first premolar on the mesial aspect and on proximal opened furcation areas on maxillary molars.

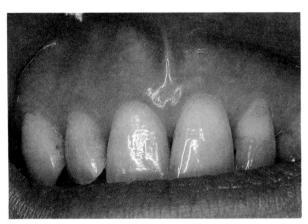

FIGURE **9–11** • Same patient 20 days after discontinuing use of tartar control toothpaste. (Courtesy Dr. Terry Rees)

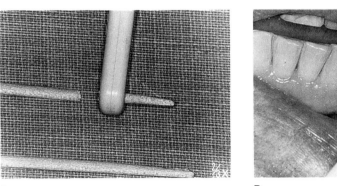

A   B

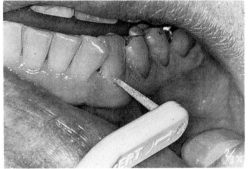

C

FIGURE **9–12** • Aids to plaque control in difficult areas. (A) Periodontal toothpick and holder (World's Fair brand). (B) Toothpick in use. The toothpick is held perpendicular to the tooth and traces the gingival margin. (C) Specialized brush (Proxybrush handle with No. 614 soft brush).

Suggestions for Teaching Plaque Control

Do not expect the patient to be perfect. Always compliment each patient before and after you show him where he is missing areas. Ask for feedback on problems, questions, and so on. Never talk down to the patient. Use several office staff members in teaching oral hygiene instructions. Individual patients may relate to one staff member better than to others.

Plaque Control Record

A cleanliness score can easily be determined after a plaque stain is used (Fig. 9–13). This positive grading system provides an incentive to the patient to do better. A graphic running record of progress (Fig. 9–14) provides further encouragement.

Bacterial Plaque Chemotherapy

A wide range of antiplaque agents have recently been introduced. This is beneficial because it makes our patients more aware of periodontal diseases and the importance of plaque control.

The only agent tested and proved to be an effective antiplaque agent to date is chlorhexidine. A commercial mouthrinse containing this substance in a 0.12% con-

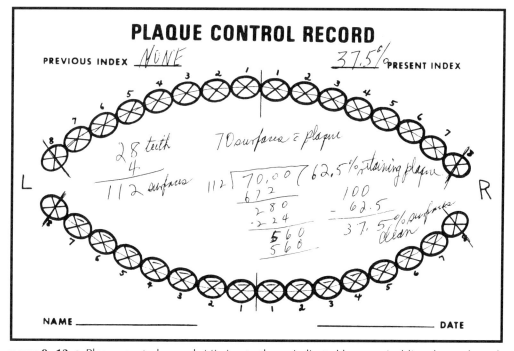

FIGURE **9–13** • Plaque control record. Missing teeth are indicated by a vertical line drawn through them. The number of teeth present is counted and multiplied by four to take account of the number of surfaces on each tooth that are in contact with the gingival margin. Dividing the number of surfaces containing plaque by the total number of surfaces yields the percentage of surfaces with plaque. This is subtracted from 100% to give the percentage of surfaces that are clean. This is the patient's cleanliness grade.

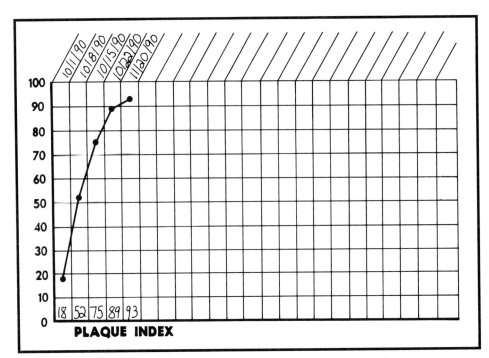

FIGURE **9–14** • Plaque index graph, showing progression in cleanliness grades over time.

centration has been approved by the Food and Drug Administration for use in patients. Chlorhexidine is very safe but can cause staining on teeth and plastics. We have found it useful as a plaque control agent after surgery and as a weekly rinse in patients who either cannot or will not practice effective plaque control.

Another chemotherapeutic plaque control method which should be mentioned because of the broad publicity it has received is the so-called Keyes technique, devised by Dr. Paul Keyes. In this method, bacterial motility is monitored microscopically and treated by various methods. The patient is instructed to use various solutions of salt, peroxide, and baking soda in pastes and water irrigators to control the plaque. When tested scientifically under controlled conditions this method was found to have little or no benefit over regular oral hygiene procedures. For this reason, and because animal studies have linked daily use of hydrogen peroxide with preneoplastic and neoplastic changes, we do not recommend this method of therapy for patient treatment.

Recall Treatment

At recall treatment, examine lips, mucous membranes, face, gingival tissues, mobility, probing, depth, and occlusion. Assess plaque control using a red-dye tablet test to determine effectiveness, and review technique with the patient.

The best treatment for incipient pockets is removal of calcified dental deposits (scaling), root planing, and curettage. If this treatment is not effective, other procedures must later be considered.

The difficult-to-maintain cases are handled by doing the following: Scale and root-plane problem areas, reoperate areas that have not responded, prescribe a 4- to 5 day course of antibiotics after each recall treatment, and extract and replace hopelessly involved individual teeth. The few patients who are most difficult to maintain should return every 2 weeks for professional plaque removal and polishing until the condition of teeth and gums is under control.

The effectiveness of a practice's recall and maintenance program is one of the primary determinants of the rate of tooth loss among patients in that practice. Therefore, the techniques used in such programs warrant detailed consideration.

No dentist can possibly care for all recall patients, so the aid of a registered dental hygienist who has been trained by the doctor in the proper techniques is essential. Hygienists should start out with a series of questions for each patient, such as: Are you having any problems in your mouth? Any discomfort from chewing, heat, or cold? Any bleeding from your gums when you brush or floss? Any bad tastes or odors? Have you been performing your plaque control twice a day? Has your health status changed? Have you any questions for the doctor?

While examining each patient the hygienist informs them what she (or he) is doing by stating, "Now I am going to check your lips, your cheeks, your tongue—would you stick it out, please, and say 'Ah'?—the floor of your mouth, your throat, and your palate." The hygienist should note any deviations from normal and bring them to the doctor's attention to evaluate. If there are no deviations, the patient should be told that everything looks beautiful. Then each tooth is checked for mobility and gingival attachment. After the hygienist first probes with her own index finger to see how much pressure is required to make the tissues blanch, she then assesses the amount of gingival deattachment with a periodontal probe. Any gingival attachments that bleed when probed lightly or have an exudate are noted (and later root planed); if the depth is over 3 mm, these areas are recorded on a new probing chart. Pockets that were 8 mm or deeper and had osseous defects before treatment will usually result in 3-mm to 4-mm crevices unless total bone repair has occurred.

Patients who smoke are reminded they need to have a yearly medical checkup. Any smoker's patches or keratotic, white, or flaky lesions on the lips, nose, and face are brought to the patient's attention, so that he (or she) can seek medical treatment.

Next, the teeth are stained to determine how effective the patient's home care regimen was in the removal of bacterial plaque. The patient is then complimented on the clean surfaces and shown the areas that have been missed. The patient is reminded of the date that the specific treatment was started and that the favorable results could have been obtained only by his good care. It should be emphasized again that a careful regimen of plaque control will be essential in order to maintain a strong foundation for the teeth and their supporting tissues in the future. When a patient has neglected plaque control, the dental hygienist shows him the neglected areas, records his oral cleanliness index, and then tells him that she will try to get all the stained plaque off before the doctor examines his mouth. This approach makes the patient feel that the hygienist is an ally and is not belittling him in any way. If surgery had originally been performed, the hygienist could tell the patient that the doctor had contoured the tissues for easier maintenance and would be extremely disappointed to see plaque on the teeth, because plaque will create new pockets later. Gracey curettes (P-7, P-8, No. 11, and No. 12), Hirschfeld files, or Orban hoes (for deep, narrow, probeable areas) are used by the hygienists supra- and subgingivally around all teeth.

The oral cleanliness index is used to record the percentage of tooth surfaces that are free of plaque. If the patient is doing an excellent job of plaque control and has plaque on only 5% of his tooth surfaces, then his oral cleanliness index is 95%.

As opposed to the O'Leary Plaque Index, which uses the percentage of tooth surfaces which do have plaque, this index gives the patient a score similar to grades in school, where higher is better. Thus, if he does poorly, he gets a 25% or 30%.

A vitalometer is used to test the vitality of symptomatic teeth. Crowned symptomatic teeth are tested for vitality with ice. Not only are the hygienists trained to test for the mobility of each tooth, they are also trained to detect fremitus of the patient's teeth while in mastication. If patients have tooth discomfort when chewing the hygienist should place sterile broad rubber bands or anesthetic rubber stoppers between the teeth, one at a time, for the patient to bite on. This will elicit pain if the patient has a split tooth. After the teeth are polished with a commercial polishing paste, the mouth is rinsed, and the hygienist flosses all contact points. Corrective and preventive recall treatments usually require a one-hour appointment for patients with a full complement of teeth.

All patients seen by the hygienist should be checked by the doctor. If any severe or serious problem is identified, an appointment is made for corrective therapy. A minor or beginning problem is cared for by the hygienist, and the next recall treatment is arranged at a shorter time interval.

Full-mouth radiographs of diagnostic quality should be taken when indicated so that bone levels, and so on, can be determined. The patient is draped with a protective lead apron and thyroid collar. For patients who are susceptible to caries, bitewing films are taken on the years that full-mouth radiographs are not. Caries-susceptible patients should also be instructed in the use of a fluoride gel for their personal care.

All patients should have an appointment in the office at all times. Following the recall treatment, make the next appointment. Patients who may later cancel are put on a standby waiting list.

Frequent recall treatments offer one of the strongest weapons for assuring treatment success and preventing tooth loss. A careful regimen of personal plaque control and professional maintenance act synergistically in the creation of a healthy periodontium.

Reappointment

Patients should be reappointed as frequently as needed before serious problems start. For some this may be 3 months and for others as much as 12 months. As a rule though, start a just-finished active treatment case an a 3-month recall. Tailor the recall interval based on the patient's oral hygiene effectiveness and disease resistance.

Failures

As with any healing arts field, one must recognize that a small proportion of the cases treated will develop new problems—further bone loss with formation of new pockets, increased mobility, and loss of individual teeth (Fig. 9–15).

One of us (CLN) surveyed 200 consecutive patients on recall in 1958 to study tooth loss. The average patient in that survey had completed active corrective treatments 4.6 years before. The average tooth loss was 0.24 teeth per person. The

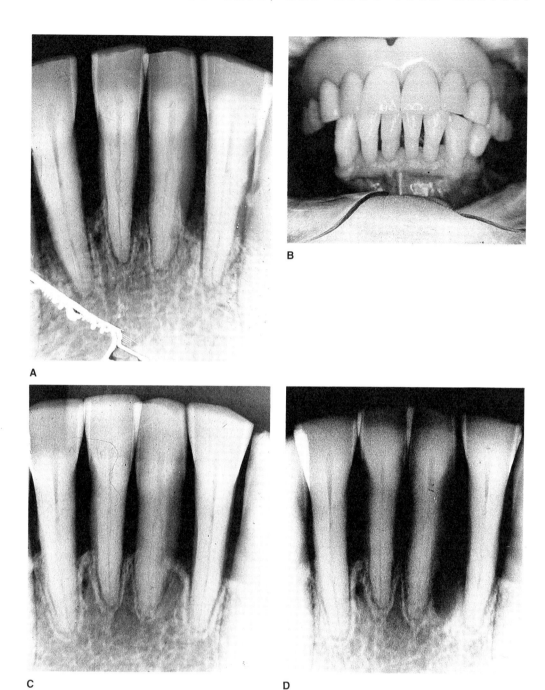

maximum tooth loss was 2. When this survey was run, four patients returned to the practice after an interval of from 1 to 7 years. These four patients had lost a total of 32 teeth in other offices, or an average of 8 teeth per person. These patients were also included in this survey. We have recently published a study which documents our practice up until 1982. In this study, 1535 patients were surveyed and the average loss remained at about the same, averaging 0.29 teeth per patient. However, 1371 patients did not lose any teeth, and the 444 teeth lost were from 164 patients. This rate of tooth loss compares favorably with other studies documenting tooth loss rates in periodontal practices. A strong, effective maintenance program has a great deal to do with the long-term success of any periodontal therapy.

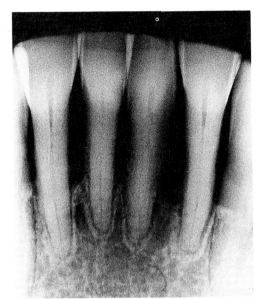

E

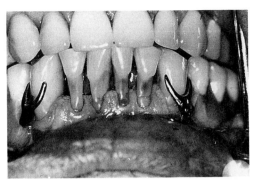

F

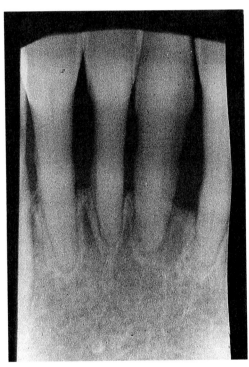

G

FIGURE **9–15** • Long-term follow-up. (*A*) Radiographic appearance at presentation. Incisors were loose and sore. Patient was wearing a full maxillary denture and a lower partial denture when first seen. She was asked to sleep without the prostheses. An apically positioned flap procedure was done. (*B*) Clinical and (*C*) radiographic appearance 2 years after surgery. (*D*) Appearance 15 years after surgery. An acute distal abscess of the central incisor was biopsied and treated by flap surgery. (*E*) Appearance 3 months later. Bone had repaired. (*F*) Clinical and (*G*) radiographic appearance 26 years after initial therapy. This was the last time the patient was seen.

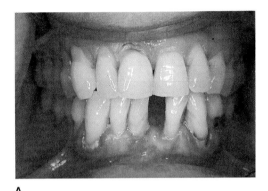

A

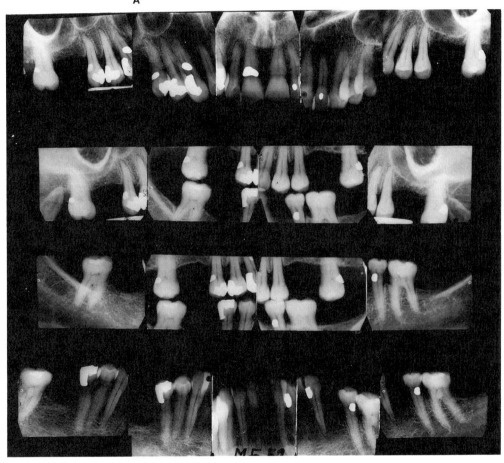

B

In spite of thorough periodontal therapy, a small number of patients will continue to lose attachment. It is now believed that this progression is due to a combination of highly pathologic bacterial strains and/or white cell defects in these patients. Tests are now available which can identify these bacteria and test antibiotic sensitivities for them. A combination of the proper antibiotic combined with thorough scalings will often halt attachment loss in refractory cases. This greatly diminishes the number of therapeutic failures. Research is now being done to test antibody responses to individual oral microorganisms. This holds the promise of further decreases in therapeutic failures.

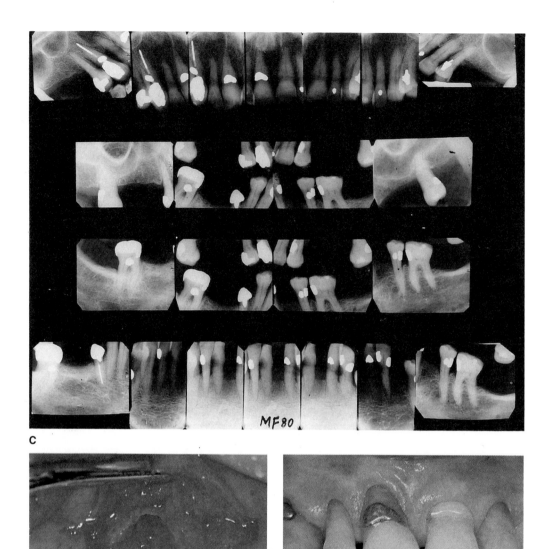

C

D   **E**

FIGURE **9–16** • Long-term follow-up. (*A*) Clinical and (*B*) radiographic appearance before treatment. (*C*) Radiographic appearance 23 years later. The patient has lost no teeth. (*D*) Periodontal abscess on the central incisor, 25 years after initial treatment. It was treated with flap surgery and root planing. (*E*) Appearance 1 year after abscess was treated. The patient died 3 years later, having lost no teeth during the 29 years she was under treatment.

Long-Term Results

When oral hygiene and follow-up procedures are properly observed, the long-term results of periodontal therapy can be gratifying to both practitioner and patient (Fig. 9–16). Within this long-term relationship, there are many vicissitudes. In some cases, stress and emotional trauma can affect oral health (Fig. 9–17). In

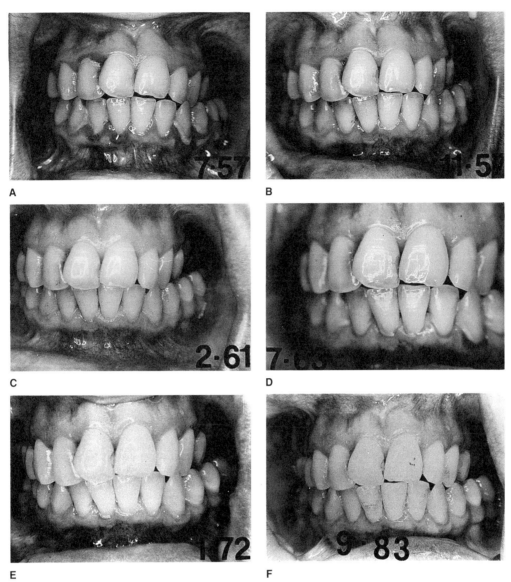

FIGURE 9–17 • Long-term follow-up. (*A*) Calculus, plaque, and gingivitis are apparent. Treatment was oral hygiene instruction and three scaling sessions. Patient was placed on a 4-month recall. (*B*) Appearance at first recall. Patient shows need for further motivation in oral hygiene. Recall was extended to 6 months after the first year. (*C*) Appearance 4 years later, before scaling. (*D*) Appearance 2 years later, a few months after the patient was told that her daughter had terminal cancer. Note poor oral hygiene and inflammation in the lower anteriors. (*E*) Appearance 8½ years later. Oral hygiene has improved. Daughter died 8 years previously. (*F*) Appearance 11 years later (26 years after *A*). Patient has been treated only by scaling, polishing, and oral hygiene motivation. (Courtesy Dr. Henry Swenson)

others, maintenance entails repeated interventions (Fig. 9–18). In yet others, comparatively minor interventions early in the relationship will suffice for long-term preservation of the dentition (Fig. 9–19). However achieved, whether by drastic intervention or continued encouragement, long-term preservation is the ideal toward which all therapy strives.

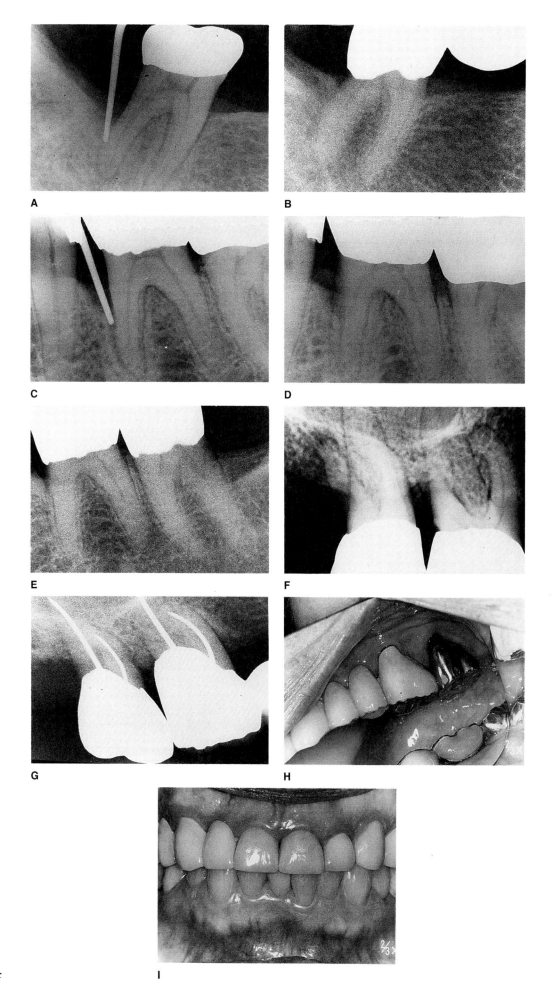

FIGURE **9–18** • Long-term follow-up. (*A*) Initial appearance of second molar. Bone grafting was done. (*B*) Appearance 23 years later. (*C*) Initial appearance of first molar, same patient. Bone grafting was also done on this tooth. (*D*) Sequestration of a portion of the graft. (*E*) Same area 24 years after surgery. (*F*) Furcation involvement, same patient. Treatment was by endodontics, distobuccal root amputations, and new crowns. The other side of the mouth required similar treatment. (*G*) Radiographic and (*H*) clinical appearance 24 years later. Note the physiologic crown contours, which allow for proper oral hygiene and physiotherapy. (*I*) Appearance 37 years after initial treatment. Patient had received regular maintenance care since complex treatment 24 years ago, and had had two reconstructions in that time.

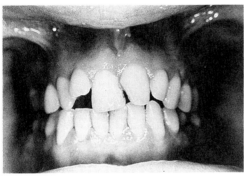
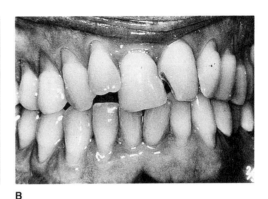

A   **B**

FIGURE **9–19** • Long-term follow-up. (*A*) Initial appearance. Beginning periodontitis is evident. Treatment was by scaling, curettage, and oral hygiene instruction. (*B*) Appearance 21 years later. Note gingival recession caused by overbrushing.

Bibliography

Axelsson P, Lindhe J. The effect of a preventive programme on dental plaque, gingivitis and caries in school children. Results after one and two years. J Clin Periodontol 1974; 1:126–138.

Breuer MM, Cosgrove RS. The relationship between gingivitis and plaque levels. J Periodontol 1989; 60:172–175.

DeVore CH, et al. Bone loss following periodontal therapy in subjects without frequent periodontal maintenance. J Periodontol 1986; 57:354–359.

Fardal O, Turnbull RS. A review of the literature on use of chlorhexidine in dentistry. J Am Dent Assoc 1986; 112:683–689.

Glavind L, et al. Oral cleanliness and gingival health following oral hygiene instruction by self-education programs. J Clin Periodontol 1984; 11:254–261.

Goldman MJ, Ross IF, Goteiner D. Effect of periodontal therapy on patients maintained for 15 years or longer. J Periodontol 1986; 57:347–353.

Grant DA, Stern IB, Everett FG. Orban's periodontics: A concept theory and practice. 4th ed. St Louis: CV Mosby, 1972.

Johansson LA, Ösfer B, Hamp SE. Evaluation of cause-related periodontal therapy and compliance with maintenance care recommendations. J Clin Periodontol 1984; 11:689–699.

Keyes PH, et al. The use of phase-contrast microscopy and chemotherapy in the diagnosis and treatment of periodontal lesions on initial report (I). Quint Int Dental Digest 1978; 9:51–56.

Lindhe J, Nyman S. Long-term maintenance of patients treated for advanced periodontal disease. J Clin Periodontol 1984; 11:504–514.

Loe H, Rindom-Schiot C. The effect of suppression of the oral microflora upon the development of dental plaque and gingivitis. In: McHugh WD, ed. Dental plaque. Edinburgh: E & S Livingston, 1970:247.

Nabers CL, Stalker WH, Esparza D, Naylor B, Canales S. Tooth loss in 1535 treated periodontal patients. J Periodontol 1988; 59:297–300.

Nyman S, Rosling B, Lindhe J. Effect of professional tooth cleaning on healing after periodontal surgery. J Clin Periodontol 1975; 2:8–86.

Nyyssonen V, Honkala E. Toothbrushing frequency in 4 consecutive studies of Finnish adolescents. J Clin Periodontol 1984; 11:682–688.

O'Leary TJ, et al. The incidence of recession in young males: A further study. J Periodontol 1971; 42:264–267.

O'Leary TJ, Nabers CL. Instructions to supplement teaching oral hygiene. J Periodontol 1969; 40:27. (These instructional booklets can be purchased from the American Academy of Periodontology, 211 East Chicago Ave, Chicago, Illinois 60611.)

O'Leary TJ, Drake RB, Naylor JE. The plaque control record. J Periodontol 1972; 43:38.

Pashley DH, Leibach JG, Horner JA. The effects of burnishing Naf/kaolin/glycerin paste on dentin permeability. J Periodontol 1987; 58:19–23.

Philstrom BL, et al. Salt and peroxide compared with conventional oral hygiene—I. Clinical results. J Periodontol 1987; 58:291–300.

Rees TD, Orth CF. Oral ulcerations with use of hydrogen peroxide. J Periodontol 1986; 57:689–692.

Soderholm G, Egelberg J. Teaching plaque control. II. 30-minute versus 15-minute appointments in a three-visit program. J Clin Periodontol 1982; 9:214–222.

Suomi JD, et al. The effect of controlled oral hygiene procedures on the progression of periodontal disease in adults: Radiographic findings. J Periodontol 1971; 42:152.

Tabita PV, Bissada NF, Maybury JE. Effectiveness of supragingival plaque control on the development of subgingival plaque and gingival inflammation in patients with moderate pocket depth. J Periodontol 1981; 52:88–93.

Van Dyke TE, Offenbacher S, Place D, Dowell VR, Jones J. Refractory periodontitis: Mixed infection with *Bacteroides gingivalis* and other unusual *Bacteroides* species—a case report. J Periodontol 1988; 59:184–189.

Waerhaug J. Effect of toothbrushing on subgingival plaque formation. J Periodontol 1981; 52:30–34.

Weitzman SA, et al. Effects of hydrogen peroxide on oral carcinogenesis in hamsters. J Periodontol 1986; 57:685–688.

Wilson TG, et al. Tooth loss in maintenance patients in a private periodontal practice. J Periodontol 1987; 58:231–235.

CHAPTER TEN

Malpractice Prevention and Periodontal Referral

Malpractice Prevention*

PATIENT RELATIONS

Emotions are the dominant force behind most malpractice claims. Patients who feel misled, betrayed, or abandoned become angry and seek vindication of their rights more than financial compensation. Therefore maintain a tactful and courteous approach and be attentive to patients' needs and complaints. Always make sure that your communications with the patient are clear, even to the point of being repetitious, by asking if the patient has any questions. Never abandon a patient in the middle of a course of treatment, and be available to provide follow-up care. Avoid telephone diagnosis, but if you must do so, make a note in the record. Good telephone communication is a matter of asking the right questions, such as asking a postoperative patient if there is difficulty in swallowing or breathing as well as the degree and location of swelling. If you are at a telephone booth, remain there until the patient calls you back with a temperature reading.

Do not make off-the-cuff diagnoses. One dentist noticed a guest's periodontal problem at a party, and it was later argued that he was responsible for damages resulting from inadequate follow-up after an encounter of mere cocktail chatter.

Keep conversations professional. Making light of a minor occurrence, like the dropping of an instrument with a quip about that "one-drink-too-many" at lunch, may not sound so funny if soberly reiterated by the patient to the jury.

---

*This section was contributed by Edwin J. Zinman, D.D.S., J.D., who is a periodontist and a practicing attorney and is one of the country's leading authorities on dental malpractice.

Young practitioners are apt to walk into unreasonable treatment traps where more experienced practitioners fear to tread. Do not let a patient's flattery of your abilities undermine your best professional judgment. Heroic measures usually result in treatment failures, a dissatisfied patient, and, ultimately, a lawsuit for uninformed consent concerning the patient's virtually hopeless prognosis.

A patient dissatisfied with prior treatment, such as a patient with a bag full of dentures or bridges made by other competent dentists, should signal a waving red flag to stop, rather than proceeding with treatment.

Good patient relations are 15% dependent upon your competency to cure and 85% upon demonstrating to the patient that you care enough to always give your professional best.

SEEK EXPERT ADVICE

Contact your insurance company or legal counsel at the first sign of serious patient discontent for advice concerning actions you can take to forestall a lawsuit by nipping a problem in the bud. Do not trivialize or ignore a patient's complaint, as this may later be construed as guilty evasion or admission by silence.

Once a suit is served, realize that you are out of your ballpark. Dentists tend to use technical dental terms as if trying to convince colleagues. But you are going to have to convince twelve lay people, so it is best to consult an attorney to translate everything into "legalese" and learn how to present a convincing public image.

One dentist was so undone that he sold his practice and took a second mortgage on his house to pay an out of court settlement fee after his insurance company refused to settle a perfectly defensible suit. A solitary malpractice suit, no matter what the outcome, rarely damages a practitioner's reputation or practice or affects future insurability.

GUARANTEES

If you guarantee treatment results which do not occur, you could be liable for breach of warranty. Frustrated expectations are the basis of many lawsuits ranging from breach of warranty to lack of informed consent. Do not promise anything other than to do your best. For instance, do not promise bonding to make a patient "look like a star."

FEES

Clarify fees and payment procedures before initiating treatment. If the dental work becomes more extensive than originally planned, discuss the increased charges and reasons with the patient before continuing treatment. Resist charging for untoward complications such as extended postoperative visits, retrieving broken instruments, or reducing unexpected fractures.

The overzealous receptionist who places payment pressure on a dissatisfied patient, or the dentist who sues to collect a fee from an already displeased patient, may invite a counter suit for malpractice. Refunding fees or paying for the treatment fee of the subsequent treating dentist under the general liability rather than professional liability portion of your policy is usually much less expensive than a week in court and a jury judgment—which also includes the intangible costs of the patient's pain and suffering. If you do sue for your fee, only do so if your treatment is beyond reproach and your records substantiate proper diagnosis and treatment and informed consent options, if applicable.

INFORMED CONSENT

The legal issue in informed consent is whether sufficient information was given to provide a reasonable patient a general understanding of the proposed treatment or procedure, including any dentally acceptable alternatives, predictable non-remote inherent risks of serious injury, and likely consequences if the patient refuses proposed therapy. Informed consent only applies to non-negligent but inherent risks of treatment, since a patient may not legally consent to negligent care. For instance, a patient who refuses necessary diagnostic radiographs should be refused treatment because a patient's consent to negligent care is legally voidable.

If a dentist fails to obtain informed consent, a plaintiff can recover damages even in the absence of any negligent treatment. Therefore, document your discussion of risks with the patient. Informed consent forms are helpful but not legally mandated. Equally, if not more, important, is a notation in the chart that you discussed informed consent risks and alternatives and the patient understood the discussion and accepted the risks. Research has shown that patients often mentally block out frightening information. Trauma and a potent anesthetic can create retrograde amnesia.

Follow only the authorized treatment plan. If an emergency precludes advising the patient of treatment risks, lack of informed consent is defensible as implied consent, since no reasonable person would refuse necessary nonelective treatment.

Record any specific treatment refused, and the patient's reason for the refusal. Patients may initial the refusal on the chart if you are extra cautious, but it is not mandatory. For example, "Patient refused orthodontic referral for consultation with Dr. Jones because husband was laid off work last month and cannot afford, but understands detrimental risk of delay."

EXPLANATIONS

Explain technical terms in lay language. A dentist who acts condescendingly and shows off his (or her) great wealth of dental knowledge creates resentment. If any future problem arises, imagined or real, the patient may not hesitate to sue.

STANDARD OF CARE

The "standard of care" is defined legally as the quality of care reasonably and prudently provided under the circumstances of treatment. Customary practice is evidence of the standard of care, but is not the exclusive determinant if the customary practice is a negligent custom. Dentists and hygienists who customarily fail to probe or take diagnostic quality radiographs, do not refer for complicated procedures beyond the ken of their training, disregard aseptic practices such as rubber gloves and face masks, and do not employ rubber dams for endodontics are typical examples of negligence.

Merely because a majority of practitioners in a community practice a particular methodology does not conclusively establish the standard of care, if such customary practice is unreasonable or imprudent. Ultimately, the courts determine reasonable dental practices, considering the available dental knowledge and the risks and benefits of a particular procedure. There is little excuse, for example, for failure to routinely probe or wear rubber gloves, irrespective of how many other dentists in the community similarly practice, since the benefit of disease recognition by probing and prevention of disease transfer by gloving outweigh the risks, which are virtually non-existent.

A lame legal defense likely to invoke a jury's wrath is to claim that a necessary diagnostic or prophylactic procedure is "time-consuming," when the failure to adopt prudent practices places the dental and medical health of the patient at risk.

In specialty categories of treatment, such as comprehensive orthodontics or advanced periodontal or full bony impaction surgery, a general practitioner will be held to the specialist's standard of care. A generalist should refer rather than perform procedures that are beyond the general practitioner's training or competency, to avoid the likely risk that a subsequent treating specialist will condemn the generalist's therapy as below the specialist's standard.

RECORD KEEPING

Records represent the single most critical evidence a dentist can present in court as a clear and accurate confirmation of diagnosis and treatment of the patient. If a dentist can only verbally refute malpractice allegations, on the basis of recall rather than records, juries will likely believe the plaintiff. For the patient, the treatment recommendations at issue are a one-time occurrence, whereas for the defending dentist the unrecorded recommendation is but one of many to large numbers of patients. Not only does a detailed record serve to substantiate an event, it sends a message to the jury that the dentist was conscientious throughout treatment, before there was any thought of a suit, and eliminates the suggestion that the dentist's recall is self-serving and selective.

Records should include a clear identification of the patient, the date of each appointment, an annually updated medical history, a comprehensive treatment plan, the patient's attitude to dentistry, the quality of the patient's home care, any patient failure to follow treatment recommendations, examination findings, laboratory prescriptions, referrals or refusals, copies of referral communications, drug prescriptions, and documentation of missed, canceled, or rescheduled appointments and payments. Evidence of patient non-compliance with instructions, such as poor plaque control or failure to seek referred treatment, can prove the patient's contributory negligence.

Abbreviated records can prove disastrous if the practitioner is unable to decipher entries during a trial. Use standard or easily understood abbreviations. Pencil entries are legally valid, but ink entries are less subject to allegations of erasure or alteration. A short pencil is still better than a long memory, since records remember but patients and dentists alike forget.

Refrain from examining records after they have been subpoenaed, to avoid anxiety and the temptation to clarify an entry. Alteration of records has become the biggest nightmare in defending cases, and a cause of large verdicts or settlements. Your records are a business document—one should not be cavalier about making changes.

To correct an entry, line out but do not erase the erroneous entry. Place and date the correction on the next available line in the chart. Handwriting and ink experts utilizing infra-red technology can prove additions, deletions or substituted records.

Records are subject to (a) audits by insurance carriers for documentation that treatment was performed; (b) review by peer review committees; and (c) subpoena by state disciplinary boards. Accordingly, incomplete or missing records expose the dentist to liability beyond professional negligence claims, such as insurance fraud.

Most juries believe a prudent dentist would be equally prudent in record keeping. To a jury, good records mean a dentist exercised his best judgment—which the law requires.

If weak records are being defended, defense attorneys often cross-examine adverse expert witnesses' records to prove that so-called good dentists also omit important findings from their records. Therefore, subpoena adverse witnesses' treating records before trial and review them with your defense attorney.

Legal proof in a civil trial requires a mere preponderance of the evidence, or a 51% tilting of the evidentary scales. That is, proof positive or absolute proof is not legally required in civil cases such as dental negligence. Consequently, when a patient at trial disputes a dentist's version of the facts, poor records are overcome with difficulty, if at all. Worst of all is altered records, which prove the dentist has not been honest with the jury and often result in inflammatory awards.

Dentists are judged in court by not only their demeanor but, more importantly, by their documented records. Few practitioners, if any, can realistically remember prior therapy, referrals, or recommendations unless they are recorded. Periodic review of the treatment plan is analogous to reviewing a road map guide to proper directions in therapy.

Good dentists with poor records have no one to blame but themselves in the event of a malpractice claim, since a prudent dentist acting in compliance with the standard of care maintains adequate dental records which document clinical findings, treatment, referrals, and recommendations.

SUPERVISED PERIODONTAL NEGLECT

Virtually all malpractice claims relating to nondiagnosis of periodontal disease gravitate about three items of proof. First, no periodontal diagnosis is recorded. Second, the chart contains no evidence of periodontal probing, not even a simple WNL (within normal limits) entry. Finally, diagnostically accurate intraoral radiographs, including repeated full-mouth radiographs every three to five years, were not taken.

Nonsurgical periodontics has emerged as both efficacious and an accepted form of periodontal therapy. As a legal defense against a charge of failing to provide pocket elimination surgery, the dentist must prove that non-surgical therapy was provided. Incomplete or nonexistent charting provides evidence of nontreatment or nonrecognition of progressive periodontitis rather than of nonsurgical care. Nonsurgical therapy is meticulous, time consuming, and technically difficult. Thus, periodontal proof of nonsurgical periodontal disease control requires documentation of probing measurements, tissue changes (including bleeding), plaque control levels, mobility, and an adequate number of diagnostic quality radiographs.

Just as one does not play golf with one club, no one exclusive method of therapy is a panacea for all patients or all quadrants. Proper periodontal therapy in the same quadrant may range from root planing to surgery or implants, if the dentist employs a diverse armamentarium and carefully selects therapy.

Patient insurance forms

An insurance form is a legal document and should be a precise and accurate reflection of the dental treatment actually delivered. Do not predate, postdate, or bill for nonexistent dental treatment. Creative billing is mailing out an invitation to be sued for fraud. Patients may request prebilling so they can be reimbursed before an insurance policy expires. Nonetheless, if the patient later becomes unhappy with the dental treatment, he may deny ever having suggested this arrangement. It is no defense that a patient requested or acquiesced in fraudulent billing: you are responsible for what is submitted. Contributory negligence of the patient is simply no defense to insurance fraud committed by the dentist.

Equipment and supplies

Keep equipment in good repair and check its condition frequently. Carefully note the manufacturer's instructions and all warnings on both medications and appliances and inform your staff. Save broken instruments or needles if a portion becomes lodged in the patient, since the manufacturer may be strictly liable rather than, or in addition to, you.

Drugs

Exercise extreme caution when using dangerous drugs and write cautionary directions on prescriptions for sedative or narcotic drugs, which the pharmacist should place on the prescription container as a patient reminder. For example, prepare a stamp which states:

> Do not drive or operate dangerous machinery after taking medication, since drowsiness is likely to occur. Alcohol and sedative or tranquilizing drugs will cause drowsiness if taken in combination with this prescribed drug.

Employees

"Vicarious negligence" is the legal principle by which a dentist is held liable for the acts and omissions of employee dentists, hygienists, or other auxiliaries. Be cautious when delegating responsibilities and give clear instructions to ensure that your staff properly represents you and your practice methods. Do not let auxiliaries practice beyond their competency level or licensed area. For example, under California law temporary restorations must be personally checked by the dentist prior to patient dismissal. Staff members should not make final diagnoses or handle patient complaints without your involvement. Instruct them to ask the appropriate questions and to relay the patient's answers to you, so that you can determine what should be done.

Registered dental hygienists should recognize dental pathology by making preliminary diagnoses subject to the dentist's final diagnosis and treatment plan.

Hygienists and dentists should routinely probe all new patients as part of a complete examination. Record periodontal pockets of 4 mm or greater depth; if none are found, indicate that a probing examination was performed but no pockets were present.

Always treat employees—even an employee you are discharging—with dignity and respect, so as not to create a desire for employee retaliation. A disgruntled employee could complain to the State Dental Board for alleged illegal practice of dentistry by auxiliaries. Document any warnings for potential discharge in the employee's personnel file, noting that if the inappropriate behavior is not corrected the employee will be discharged. Sudden, on-the-spot firing without providing an opportunity for corrective behavior may subject the employer dentist to a suit for wrongful termination and a claim for punitive damages.

KEEP CURRENT

Read dental literature and take pertinent Continuing Education courses so that you are confident of offering the most current clinically acceptable treatment. Do not be the first or the last to adopt new techniques or devices.

Avoid blind acceptance of every new technique. Refer to the American Dentistry Association's toll-free number (800-621-8099 or 800-621-3291) when you have doubts about the legitimacy of any methodology or desire information about sterilization to prevent AIDS or hepatitis transmission.

Be prepared to deal with the risks of dangerous undertakings. The most substantial settlements and jury awards involve untreated periodontitis, defective crowns and bridges, anesthesia, infection, cancer, nerve injuries, and hemorrhages. Most frequently litigated are claims concerning non-recognition, treatment of referral of periodontitis, defective crowns, and inadequate endodontics. Punitive damages have been awarded in cases where the crown margins were grossly open but crowns were knowingly cemented anyway.

REFERRALS

Develop a reliable referral network for patient personality types or treatment plans with which you are uneasy. Refer if difficulties arise or persist after initial treatment. If you notice any unusual symptom, consult the patient's personal physician or refer to an appropriate dental specialist.

Some dentists hesitate to advise a patient to obtain a second opinion or refer to a specialist for fear of arousing suspicions of incompetence or feelings of abandonment. On the contrary, the patient's trust is usually strengthened when they are given such attention. No single dentist is capable of doing all procedures necessary under every circumstance for every patient. Specialists also have a duty to refer problems that are beyond their ken. The law does not require 100% perfection or ideal dentistry but rather reasonable competency.

Communicate the patient's condition directly to the referred doctor in specific terms, both verbally and in writing. Identify the specific teeth for treatment both by the universal system and also by diagram to avoid confusion. If the patient refuses the referral, document the reason for refusal and then give serious thought to whether you desire to continue treatment. Before any treatment has begun, a dentist may decline to treat a patient who refuses a referral.

Rapport

The better the rapport is between dentist and patient the less likely is the patient to sue. Develop rapport by demonstrating genuine interest in the patient and making the patient feel like the most valued patient in the practice.

Patients feel important if seated within a reasonable time after arrival. The longer the waiting period the greater will be the patient's frustration and animosity. If the patient cannot be seen within a reasonable time, a staff member should communicate the reason and if appropriate offer a reappointment. Staff or doctor should telephone the patient at the end of the day following any difficult procedure or surgery as a reminder to follow postoperative instructions. Record any patient noncompliance.

Previous dentist's treatment

Do not be overprotective of blatant examples of substandard dental treatment. If you do discover a gross violation of the minimum standard of dental care, you have an ethical responsibility to report the matter to your local dental society peer review board and/or the Board of Dental Examiners. If you do not, and the patient later learns that he or she suffers from poor treatment, then technically you could be sued as a co-conspirator to fraudulent concealment of another practitioner's neglect. Corroborate your suspicion of prior care deficiencies by obtaining the patient's authorization for transfer of a copy of the prior dentist's records, including radiographs. Also consider speaking with the prior dentist to obtain his or her view of what occurred.

Treatment complications

Untoward results should be discussed with patients no matter how unlikely further complications or patient discovery of the problem may seem. In a court of law, a failure to disclose an unfavorable outcome is considered concealment or suppression of material facts tantamount to fraud. Discontinuing treatment in the presence of complications is abandonment. Treat to completion or refer.

Be honest and advise the patient of an adverse or unexpected result. Take control of the situation by administering or referring for proper corrective action. There is nothing wrong with saying you are sorry, which is only an admission of human compassion rather than guilt.

A patient who is never informed of an untoward result feels betrayed. For instance, a dentist may worry that the patient will be horrified to discover that an endodontic instrument fractured. However, a bad result alone is not negligence. It may happen despite the best of care, which is the distinction between a maloccurrence and malpractice. Thus, a broken-instrument case is often defensible if the patient was advised of the fracture. Save the broken end of the instrument, whether it be reamer or needle, since the cause of the fracture may be a defect in the product for which the manufacturer is strictly liable.

Exercise caution when billing a patient who has experienced an unsatisfactory outcome. A disappointed but otherwise understanding patient may feel that insult has been added to injury and elect to file suit. Most dentists are unaware that treatment complications are covered under the Medical Payments provision of professional liability policies for "accidents." Payment up to $500 and sometimes more may be provided for subsequent treatment by a physician or a dental specialist, or any other reasonable medical or dental expense. No malpractice claim should be recorded against your malpractice policy or record, since "medical payment" reimbursement falls under the general liability rather than the professional liability provision of your policy.

LIABILITY INSURANCE

It is currently recommended that a dentist acquire a minimum of $1 million worth of malpractice protection. Add excess coverage if you routinely perform hospital treatment. Do not practice with an underinsured dentist, especially if you are in a partnership, as opposed to a corporation, or you may be held liable for the underinsured dentist's damages. The "deep pocket" theory of joint and several liability allows the court in some states to assess damages against the person with the most coverage, regardless of the amount of responsibility, if the co-defendent is underinsured or judgment-proof.

Purchase an occurrence-type policy, in which you are covered forever for treatment delivered during the year you were insured, even if you are sued years later. With a claims-made policy, you must be insured the same year you are sued—which occurs infrequently since claims are usually filed when discovered years later. Extended coverage, or "tail" endorsement, may be available, but some practitioners retire and neglect to purchase this coverage or advise the spouse to purchase it if the dentist should predecease the spouse. Unexpectedly, years later, the dentist or surviving spouse is sued for dental treatment performed or omitted 20 years earlier and there is no coverage. In addition, tail coverage may not always be available if the current carrier withdraws from the market or the dentist changes carriers.

Insurance companies prefer claims-made policies because of the volatility of the malpractice climate. Such policies are initially less expensive for the dentist and more economically feasible for the company, which charges premiums on projected claims assessments. Claims-made policies offer limited protection for only the year of purchase and do not offer a continuing coverage in the absence of an additional premium for tail coverage.

CONCLUSION

The Platinum Rule is to do unto your patients as they would have done unto themselves. Treating the patient's best interest serves the best interests of the dental profession and, consequently, the dental practitioner. Conversely, treating only the dentist's financial interest by treatment designed to plunder the patient's insurance company is contrary to the standard of care and subjects the dentist to a fraud suit for punitive damages. Insurance carriers will only pay negligence damages, not fraud, since negligence is inadvertent, whereas fraud is intentional.

Do not be a good dentist caught with poor records at trial since juries righteously and rightfully believe that good dentists and their staffs maintain good records.

Remember the Basic 3 R's of malpractice prevention: *records, records,* and *records.*

The professional life you save may be your own. Good dentists with good records have little to fear about being successfully sued, even in the 90's.

When and Why Refer Periodontal Patients?

Referral to a periodontist must be considered in any of the following circumstances:

1. You have no interest in treating periodontal pathosis of any kind and want to refer all periodontal patients.
2. The patient's periodontal involvement is more extensive than you feel competent to treat.
3. The prognosis on a case is so doubtful or poor that you want to share this responsibility with a periodontist experienced in treating advanced cases.
4. You have reserved so much time for your own specialty (crowns, bridges, partials, etc.) that you truly do not have the time to spend doing thorough periodontal therapy.
5. Treatment results are less than acceptable and the wise course of action is to refer the patient to a periodontist. Hanging in there and not referring the patient can lead to legal problems if and when this patient moves to another dentist or leaves your city.

What should a referring doctor look for in a periodontist? These are important considerations:

1. Does the periodontist treat your patients as well as you expect and in the manner you would want to be treated?
2. Do your patients return and thank you for referring them to the periodontist?
3. Does your philosophy of treatment agree with the periodontist's?
4. Does the periodontist tell your patient that you are an outstanding doctor and were alert in recognizing the problems when treatment was still possible?
5. When you and Dr. X have a difference of opinion can you always arrange a consultation with him by telephone or in one of the offices or at a breakfast or lunch meeting to discuss what is best for the patient? NOTE: It is advisable to get to know your periodontist so that you can get the best combined therapy result possible for each patient. Patients are always happy to know that you and your periodontist have arranged to get together to discuss their case.
6. It is sometimes necessary to have more than one periodontist to refer to. For example your observations may have shown that one periodontist treats cases of some types better than another periodontist and vice versa.

How To Refer Periodontal Patients

The following narrative, contributed by Dr. Dalton Connor, is presented as an illustration of how referral decisions are made.

Consultation with some of my best referral sources on how best to refer a patient to a periodontist, in combination with my own experiences in receiving new patients, yields three major areas of consideration:

1. The general practitioner should diagnose the condition, educate the patient, and initiate treatment whenever possible in order to establish in the patient's mind confidence in his doctor's awareness and knowledge of periodontics. This sets the foundation for a successful referral.
2. The referring doctor should transfer the patient's confidence to the periodontist. The generalist can inform the patient that he has helped him with his periodontal condition to the extent of his skill and knowledge and that he is now in need of specialized treatment. Tell the patient who you want him to see and why. It is important in the transfer of confidence to another office to recommend only one periodontist and to tell the patient why you recommend that person. An effective statement to support your recommendation could be, "If I had your problem I would want Dr. _X_ to be my periodontist." Avoid discussion of anticipated periodontal treatment or costs. This tends to create unnecessary fears that can disrupt the referral process. Just simply state the problem as you see it, potential disadvantages to anticipate if not treated, and how much there is to be gained if successfully managed. Tell the patient: "Let Dr. _X_ thoroughly examine you, and listen to his recommendations." Let the patient and periodontist know your primary areas of concern, but try not to limit your periodontist's examination to a specific area since this can become a source of embarrassment if other potential problems are noted.
3. Communication should be maintained between referring doctor and periodontist. Most doctors want to be kept informed about the status of their patients by letter, telephone, or both. It is also important for the periodontist to learn from the referring doctor what treatment has been done, the patients' response and attitude, restorative objective, and any other information that can help in making treatment decisions. When you and your patient choose a periodontist you are inviting him or her to be a member of your treatment team. Therefore, the flow of information must go in both directions.

There is certainly room for extensive and valuable discussion on this subject of how to refer a patient. However, serious attention to the above basic principles should aid the referral process.

Bibliography

Emphasis: Professional liability: Has the crisis passed? J Am Dent Assoc 1988; 116:470–478.

Zinman EJ. Advise before you incise. J West Soc Periodontol 1976.

Zinman EJ. Usual and customary versus prudent practice. J Tennessee Dent Assoc 1979; 60-3:9–13.

Dental Records
Sample record charts, including informed consent, may be obtained by sending $5 to:
Wisconsin Dental Association
633 West Wisconsin Avenue
Milwaukee, Wisconsin 53202

Index